25

Biomechanics
of running shoes

Edited by
Benno M. Nigg, Dr. sc. nat.
University of Calgary

Human Kinetics Publishers, Inc.
Champaign, Illinois

Library of Congress Cataloging in Publication Data
Main entry under title:

Biomechanics of running shoes.

Bibliography: p.
Includes index.
1. Running shoes. 2. Running. 3. Foot. 4. Human
mechanics. I. Nigg, Benno Maurus.
TS1017.B56 1986 685'.36 85-2460
ISBN 0-87322-002-1

Developmental editor: Sue Wilmoth, PhD
Production director: Sara Chilton
Copy editor: Olga Murphy
Typesetter: Sandra Meier
Layout artist: Lezli Harris
Printed by: Edwards Brothers

9 8 7 6 5 4 3 2 1

ISBN: 0-87322-002-1

Human Kinetics Publishers, Inc.
Box 5076, Champaign, IL 61820

Acknowledgments

A project of this size cannot be done without two major groups of support: the support of colleagues and co-workers, and the support of institutions. It is not only an obligation but also a desire for me to acknowledge this support in mentioning the most important individuals and institutions, which are as follows:

Adidas sport shoe manufacturers (H. Dassler & W. Anderie) provided many sets of special shoes that were used for the systematic studies. These shoes were specially constructed so that everything was identical except the one aspect that was studied in-depth. Furthermore, since 1977, this company has financially supported, and continues to support, the various research projects. I am very pleased that Adidas is prepared to invest money in the basic research of running shoes, and that they promote the publication of the results so that every runner can profit from the information.

Nike sport shoe manufacturers (E.C. Frederick & T. Clarke) have financially supported our research in the field of sport shoes since 1982. They were always prepared to exchange ideas in methodology and in application. The mutual discussions initiated several new ideas on how to experiment in the field of sport shoe analysis.

The Swiss National Foundation for Research for many years supported a project which dealt with the basic analysis of load on the locomotor system and the mathematical modelling of it. This project is one of the foundations on which our approach in load analysis and sport shoe research is based. In the beginning many aspects were not clear at all but are now better understood because of this support.

The ETH Zurich (Director E. Freitag) provided support for measuring equipment and computers used in the various projects, supported the continuous development of the Biomechanics Laboratory in Zurich, and provided the financial background for such a research group and, consequently, for this special project of the analysis of running shoes.

The Alberta Heritage Foundation for Medical Research allowed with its Establishment Grant the development of the Biomechanics Laboratory of the University of Calgary. It is obvious that research with respect to load on the human body in running and studies analyzing the possibilities how these forces can be controlled and reduced has a very strong medical component in it. It is probably more effective to prevent injuries instead of healing them. Our research with running and running shoes has its goal exactly in this preventive medical field in reducing forces on the human body. Therefore, I am convinced that we fulfill one of the goals of this Foundation to do research which can be applied from a medical point of view.

The Natural Sciences and Engineering Research Council of Canada (NSERC) supported and continues to support a project on impact forces during running. This project enables us to comprehensively investigate the basic factors influencing impact forces in running. It allows an approach from an engineering point of view and adds another dimension to the medical approach of running injury analysis.

The University of Calgary in 1980 decided to support research in sport science and provide the necessary infrastructure for it. In doing so, they provided the basic conditions for the development of the Biomechanics Laboratory of this University and created the environment for our research in the field of running shoes.

The Faculty of Physical Education of the University of Calgary (Dean Roger Jackson) actively supported the development of this new research unit and all the activities connected with it. They provided financial support for the additional equipment and created an outstanding environment for research activity. Many of the findings presented in the experimental part of this book are from research performed in this unit and illustrate the outstanding contribution of the Faculty of Physical Education in this context.

The list of the main supporters illustrates the dimension of the project, and I am pleased to be able to express my gratitude and appreciation to these sponsors. I hope that these supporters will accept part of our appreciation in the form of this publication.

As I put together the final version of this book, for the sake of interest, I tried to add up the people who contributed in a significant way. This summary, which does not claim to be complete, showed that in addition to the authors, 16 co-workers and technical staff, and 23 graduate students were significantly involved in the final product. These numbers are a conservative estimation, however.

To name all these co-workers is not possible. However, I would like to mention a few whose contributions were exceptional. Our first measurements were basically mechanical in approach. We measured acceleration and tried to give a mechanical interpretation of the results. However, we soon realized that such an isolated approach could not provide a comprehensive answer to the problems connected with running and running injuries. In searching for a medical counterpart, we found Dr. Bernhard Segesser, a physician who spent days and weeks cooperating with us and opening our eyes to the medical, physiological, and anatomical aspect of our research. His extensive knowledge on sport injuries and his interest in our work were important factors responsible for our development in this area. Dr. Segesser's interest in the translation of our results into the clinical situation was an important stimulus to continue our work.

Furthermore, I would like to thank Edgar Stuessi, the current Director of the Biomechanics Laboratory at the ETH, Zurich. When I moved to Calgary, he made it possible to establish cooperation between the two groups, Zurich and Calgary—which resulted in this book. Due to his generosity and his initiative, this project was developed to this level.

I also feel very thankful to Edith Unold and Xaver Kaelin, two research fellows of the Biomechanics Laboratory, ETH, Zurich. They were involved (Edith since 1972 and Xaver since 1980) in most of the projects in the running shoe studies and contributed significantly to the outcome of these projects. In addition, I feel indebted to Veronica Fisher, Louise Beauchamp, and Jim Burrett, technicians at the Biomechanics Laboratory of the University of Calgary, who helped develop the laboratory and were heavily involved in most of the projects of the last 3 years.

First, an additional thanks goes to Rosie Neil and Bettina Bahlsen for the careful preparation of the graphs. Also to type such a book and to read the handwriting of some of the authors (especially mine) is a special task. However, the cooperation with Marjorie Foofat (who did the majority of the typing), and Barbara Lees (who was very much involved in the typing of the mathematical equations) was a pleasure. They worked diligently to make our sentences sound like English.

Benno M. Nigg

Contents

Preface

A runner who wants to buy a pair of running shoes is confronted with a wide range of models, ranging from inexpensive to expensive, from soft to hard, and from red to yellow. These shoes may have special features like wedges or exchangeable damping elements which visually underline the special quality of the shoe. Advertisements for running shoes in runner's magazines explain their products by using words such as "support," "rearfoot control," "cushioning," "shock distributor," and "heel stabilizer." Although these expressions were not used in the early seventies, they are very familiar to the average runner today. Obviously, *somebody* has been thinking about the special aspects of running shoe construction. Thus, we can assume that the shoes on the market in the mid-eighties are better than the shoes a runner was able to buy in the early seventies.

One aspect of running shoe design is the protection and/or the reduction of injuries. In other words, it is the aspect of forces acting on the human body, and also the effects these forces produce in this system. During the last 10 to 15 years, research groups in the field of sport biomechanics have studied these aspects. The authors of this book represent two groups involved in this research with running shoes. The research sites are located in the Biomechanics Laboratory of the ETH in Zurich (Switzerland) and, since 1981, in the Biomechanics Laboratory of the University of Calgary (Canada). Research in sport shoes started in 1972 with a project in Zurich which included various types of sport shoes and playing surfaces. The project was a reaction to the comments from the sport medical community that so-called "hard" surfaces were generating new types of sport injuries or increasing the frequency of already known injuries.

In the following years, this initial project evolved into two main branches: one connected with playing surfaces, and the other with sport shoes, especially running shoes. Thirteen years have passed since the beginning of this project, and so it seems appropriate to present our group's most important findings of the research with running shoes. This book, therefore, will summarize and synthesize the work of these two research groups.

However, the biomechanics laboratories of the ETH, Zurich, and of the University of Calgary were not the only groups working in the field of running shoe research and running injury analysis. Outstanding work has also been performed by the biomechanics laboratory of The Pennsylvania State University with Peter Cavanagh and his co-workers, the Nike Sport Research Laboratory with Ned Frederick and his co-workers, and several other laboratories in the sport biomechanics field. Injury analysis was done by Segesser in Basel, Clement and co-workers in Vancouver, James and co-workers in Eugene, and many other sport medical specialists. Our work was greatly influenced and enriched by results and impulses from these groups and by controversies with them. Although it emphasizes our results, the organization of this book allows an overview of and a comparison with the findings of these groups and of our own.

Attempting to summarize and synthesize the research of a decade presented several difficulties. One of the problems was that many aspects of the research are theoretical, and not every reader would want to read about theory. As a result, we decided to write the book for anyone who would like to know more about running shoes, and also for anyone interested in the "behind the scenes" connections.

The theoretical ideas, the assumptions, and the calculations are described in special chapters so that only those who are interested can study these sections; those who are not can leave theory aside and go to the next chapter. These theoretical considerations, however, were included because we think that further advancement in biomechanical research with respect to running shoes lies greatly in the development of theoretical solutions.

Thus, this book is intended equally for those connected with research in running shoes; for those involved with the production or distribution of running shoes; and/or for just those who use running shoes and want to know what shoe to buy and why.

In the first chapter, Benno Nigg explains the purpose of the research and its philosophical justification with special emphasis on load on the human body. The chapter then deals with special aspects of load, underlines the influence of the geometrical and time aspects of load, and explains the concept of impact and active forces. This concept is important, and we use it in all our research and apply it throughout the book.

The second chapter (Nigg) provides an overview of the experimental measuring techniques used in connection with running shoe analysis. Force platform analysis with force, center of pressure, and moment of rotation measurements is described; pressure distribution measurements which were developed mainly for running shoes by the Penn State group are also discussed. Another major part of this chapter deals with film and film analysis and the methodology which was developed by our group. Furthermore, friction measurements are explained, and a short section deals with material tests, in particular, drop tests. Our group has many reservations in respect to these material tests, and these reservations are repeated and supported by many results throughout the book. The experimental methods have one important general aspect which is discussed for force and film—the selection of the variables which are used for running shoe analysis. This aspect is important and deserves to be presented in depth.

In the third chapter Jachen Denoth discusses the possibilities and problems of using models in running shoe analysis. Undoubtedly, the knowledge of internal forces or stresses provides much useful information in connection with load, running injuries, and running shoes. However, the determination or estimation of these quantities is not simple. Thus, it is not surprising that this chapter is the most theoretical one, presenting many unsolved questions and focusing on the critical problems of running shoe research in the last decade.

In chapter 4, Alex Stacoff and Simon Luethi describe aspects of the "anatomy" of the running shoe and of the human foot. Understanding these boundary conditions is critically important in running and running shoe analysis. The geometrical arrangement of the anatomical structures in the foot and the geometry of the running shoe are influencing the transfer from external to internal forces. Therefore, it is helpful to have some idea about the various possibilities to include in theoretical and/or experimental consideratons.

The authors of chapter 5 (Nigg, Bahlsen, Denoth, Luethi, & Stacoff) summarize a large number of experiments conducted in the last 13 years and include many ideas from members (not specifically identified) of these two groups. Whenever possible, the results are summarized generally, assuming that some of the aspects are quite well understood. In many special cases, the combination of results of various subprojects did provide support of speculations on hypotheses made in other connections.

Research in running shoes is certainly applied research. Our book would be incomplete if these findings would not be translated into the practical everyday situation of a runner. This is done in chapter 6, providing some comments for the runner in respect to the question, "Which is the best shoe?" Of course, this chapter will not produce a 5-star rating system; however, it does discuss the important factors to consider in buying a running shoe, and also explains how movement can be controlled in order to reduce the probability of a running injury.

Contributing Authors

(In alphabetical order)

Alexander H. Bahlsen
Biomechanics Laboratory
University of Calgary
Calgary, Alberta, Canada

Jachen Denoth
Laboratorium für Biomechanik
ETH Zürich
Zürich, Switzerland

Simon M. Luethi
Biomechanics Laboratory
University of Calgary
Calgary, Alberta, Canada

Benno M. Nigg
Biomechanics Laboratory
University of Calgary
Calgary, Alberta, Canada

Alex Stacoff
Laboratorium für Biomechanik
ETH Zürich
Zürich, Switzerland

1

BENNO M. NIGG

Biomechanical aspects of running

The human body is *not* constructed to sit in an office chair all day long. For normal health to be maintained, the cardiorespiratory and locomotor systems must be regularly stimulated. Increasing inactivity in the work place has, for many people, resulted in an almost subconscious drive to be more active during their free time. Since Turnvater Jahn promoted physical activities in Germany in the last century, sport, especially leisure-time sport, has become increasingly important in a person's life. This is also true for many sport activities, such as tennis, volleyball, soccer, and, of course, running and jogging. Only 20 years ago, people running or jogging in parks or on streets were considered as being outsiders. However, in these 20 years, the number of joggers has increased drastically as illustrated in Figure 1.1 (Krissoff & Ferris, 1979). Cavanagh (1980) comments that "some authorities put the number of people in the United States who run regularly at more than thirty million" which means that more than every tenth American is infected by this "jogging virus." Runners and joggers appear not only in advertisements for vitamins and sport clothes, but also for goods like cars, houses, and so on. The outsider of the 1960s is now "in" because running is "healthful, fun, and chic" (*The Physician and Sportsmedicine*, December 1979).

Furthermore, this development is illustrated by the number of popular books published about running and jogging. In addition to that, since 1970, the number of scientific publications connected with sportshoes and playing surfaces has been higher than ever before. *A Bibliography of Biomechanics Literature* (Hay, 1981) cites 5 publications on sport footwear before and 18 after 1970; 3 before versus 17 after 1970 on playing sur-

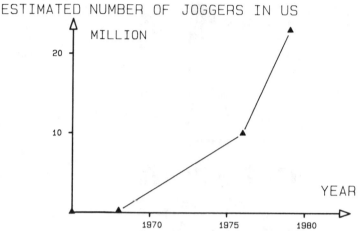

Figure 1.1. Estimated number of joggers in the United States (Krissoff & Ferris, 1979).

faces. Many of these publications, the popular as well as the scientific ones, discuss injuries and pain connected with different sport activities.

A *Runner's World* survey in 1977 stated that two out of three joggers were affected by injuries each year. The most frequent injuries are (Krissoff & Ferris, 1979) knee injuries (25%), including chondromalacia, patellar compression syndrome, patellar tendinitis, iliotibial band friction syndrome, fat pad inflammation, popliteus tendinitis, pes bursitis, gastrocnemius tendinitis or bursitis, medial retinacular inflammation, chronic instabilities, and arthritis. The second most common injury is Achilles tendinitis (18%). Shin splint is the third most common injury reported with 15%. Cavanagh (1980), using reports from *Runner's World* surveys as well as from a clinical survey, states that between 1973 and 1977 "the percentage of runners getting injured did not change appreciably in the four years between surveys." However, he reads from the statistics that the following four categories of injuries show considerable increases between 1971 and 1979:

- Leg fractures
- Heel spur syndromes
- Shin splints
- Knee injuries

Cavanagh credits the increasing number of the first three injury types to the improved diagnostic methods, while he admits that the increasing number of knee injuries is realistic and "give genuine cause for worry." However, he states that Achilles tendinitis dropped by about 10% in the period between 1971 to 1979. It is interesting that similar results were found in tennis (Nigg & Denoth, 1980). In an analysis of 1,003 tennis players, more than 50% of them indicated injuries. (Note that *injury* in this context is defined as impairment of the locomotor system which

Table 1.1. Order of magnitude of the occurrence of injuries depending on site (only steps of 5% used for the relative frequency).

Site	Relative frequency (%)	Range of relative frequency (%)
Knee	30	18 - 42
Tibia	15	10 - 20
Achilles tendon	10	6 - 20
Arch	10	7 - 14
Others	35	22 - 46

reduces the level of normal sports activity. The expressions *injury* or *pain and injury* will be used in this sense in the following.)

A summary of injuries with respect to *site* can be compiled by using the results of questionnaire studies (*Runner's World*, 1971, 1973) or the results of clinical studies (Brubaker & James, 1974; James, Bates, & Osternig, 1978; Krissoff & Ferris, 1979; Smith, 1979; Cavanagh, 1980; Pagliano & Jackson, 1980; Clement, Taunton, Smart, & McNicol, 1981). These studies show an average occurrence of pain and/or injuries as found in Table 1.1.

The results of these studies reporting injury frequencies can be discussed as follows:

1. The most frequent site for running injuries is the knee. A subdivision of the results based on the year of publication of the studies indicates that these knee injuries seem to have increased over the period between 1971 and 1981 (see Figure 1.2). Based on the reported results,

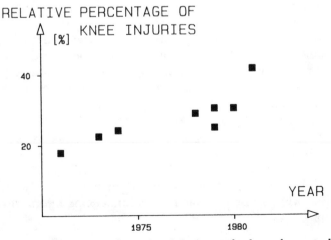

Figure 1.2. Relative number of running injuries at the knee from studies between 1971 and 1981.

it cannot be concluded whether this result is connected with different diagnosis techniques or whether it is a fact. However, it is speculated that these numbers reflect a real trend.

2. Problems at the tibia have the second highest frequency of occurrence. They include *shin splint* which is defined by the *American Medical Association's Standard Nomenclature of Athletic Injuries* as "pain and discomfort in the leg from repetitive running on hard surfaces or forcible extensive use of the foot flexors. . . . The diagnosis should be limited to musculotendinous inflammation, excluding a fatigue fracture or ischemic disorder." However, Jackson (1978) states that this definition "is not widely accepted in athletic circles." It is a form of pain or soreness at the shin which is usually present at the beginning of a workout period. The etiology of shin splint is still not absolutely clear (actually there are multiple etiologies).

3. There seems to be a tendency that the occurrence of Achilles tendon problems is decreasing since the early 1970s. The change in shoe construction has possibly had an influence as suggested by Cavanagh (1980).

4. It is quite interesting that the reason for the positive change in the frequency of Achilles tendon problems is assigned to the shoe but that no such comment is found in the literature for the increased frequency of knee and shin splint problems.

5. All the publications used in this context are from North America. Similar studies with corresponding results for running and jogging were not found in the European literature. However, it may be that statistics in Europe show different results because running habits may differ compared to North America (e.g., more running on streets in North America as compared to Europe).

6. We do not have any knowledge of similar statistics of the normal population. It may well be that in certain categories of injuries, the results of such a "normal population" statistic would not differ from the results summarized here. However, it is speculated that some of the injuries are typical for running (e.g., shin splint, knee pain) and that they would show a significantly higher frequency of occurrence in the running population.

These facts and speculations indicate that some of the "healthy activities" are not without problems. Therefore, it appears worthwhile to reflect on the possible causes for such injuries. Once again, during a year of running, two out of three joggers or runners will most likely have an injury which reduces or prevents their normal activity. The following paragraphs will discuss possible factors influencing injuries in jogging or running.

Factors Influencing Jogging and Running Injuries

Some authors suggest that certain types of *surfaces* are the origin of such injuries. The first critical publications came from medical doctors (Segesser, 1970; Prokop, 1972; Hess & Hort, 1973), who reported observations connected with the "new" type of pain and injuries they were finding in athletes with heavy training load on artificial surfaces. Several other publications based on medical observations followed (Hort, 1976; Prokop, 1976; Segesser, 1976; Bolliger, 1979). A few years after the first medical concerns about surfaces were voiced, publications of biomechanical measurements appeared, describing acceleration, force, and impact measurements on different types of surfaces (Unold, 1974; Nigg, Neukomm, & Unold, 1974; Bowers & Martin, 1974; Denoth, 1977; Nigg, Denoth, Neukomm, & Segesser, 1978; Bates, Osternig, Mason, & James 1979). The general comments were that the impact forces at first contact with the surface are higher on most of the artificial surfaces than on natural surfaces (e.g., grass), and that most of the artificial surfaces are not likely to allow any sliding and show a considerably higher resistance against rotation. Statistics published for football players (Bramwell et al., 1972) as well as tennis players (Nigg & Denoth, 1980) also support the idea that the surface may be the origin of these injuries.

Other studies consider the construction of the running *shoe* as a possible factor influencing the occurrence of injuries. These studies indicate that the shoe should protect the foot and the locomotor system against impact forces which are too high and should provide stability for the foot (Nigg, Eberle, Frey, & Segesser, 1977; Subotnick, 1979; Cavanagh & Lafortune, 1980; Smart, Taunton, & Clement, 1980; Clarke, Frederick, & Cooper, 1983; Clarke, Frederick, & Hamill, 1984; Nigg et al., 1984). Considerable evidence suggests that shoe construction and injuries are connected and that orthotic foot support should help to reduce existing pain or to reduce the development of pain and injuries (Nigg et al., 1977; Nigg et al., 1978; Segesser, Ruepp, & Nigg, 1978; Hort, 1979; Cavanagh, 1980; Segesser & Nigg, 1980; Nigg et al., 1982; Clement, 1982). The drastic development of running was probably the reason for including five laboratory tests in the *Runner's World* annual shoe survey and for expanding to eight tests in 1980 (Cavanagh, 1980). The *Runner's World* test attempted to offer guidance in shoe selection among the increasing number of different shoes by providing the consumer with "hard facts".

Some authors stressed that the interaction between *shoe and surface* is important (Unold, 1974; Bonstingel, Morehouse, & Niebel, 1975; Rheinstein, Morehouse, & Niebel, 1978), and this aspect has now become well accepted.

Another factor describing the etiology of running injuries is the type of *movement* (Nigg et al., 1978). It was proposed that a comprehensive analysis of load on the locomotor system should include the velocity of contact, the geometry of the human body at contact, and the type of movement. Furthermore, the number of repetitions which may be roughly considered equivalent to the number of kilometers an athlete runs during a week has to be included. James et al. (1978) connected about 60% of all the running injuries with the type of training of the injured athlete. The mileage per week and the intensity of the training interval were the main factors determining the ocurrence of pain.

Clement et al. (1981) found overpronation to be one of the important factors connected with running injuries. Various examples of pronation during ground contact are illustrated in Figure 1.3. The left example shows a subject with heavy pronation (overpronation); the example in the center shows another subject with very little pronation; and the example on the right illustrates a third subject who remains on the outside of the foot during the whole contact, having very little pronatory movement. The examples illustrated are not equally frequent in the running population. The example on the right side seldom occurs (probably less than 1%). The example on the left side (overpronation) is more frequent. Most of the subjects are between heavy overpronation and very little pronation when running with running shoes.

It is interesting that studies of the various factors—surface, shoe, and movement—appear clustered geographically as well as chronologically. Publications on surfaces were mainly found in Europe in the early 1970s. Publications on shoes in connection with running injuries started a few years later in Europe as well as in North America. Studies in which the movement is the main concern only started in the late 1970s and are still in the minority.

Important Aspects of a Running Shoe

"The most important piece of equipment a runner has is his shoes," wrote Bob Anderson, the editor of *Runner's World*, in 1975, and he repeated it in other editions of this magazine. A great percentage of runners may agree with this statement, and it seems evident that it is correct. However, the selection of a new pair of running shoes may depend on health, financial status, or on other factors. Different aspects must be taken into consideration. The final outcome depends on various factors, some of which are listed in Figure 1.4. The list of important aspects may look somewhat different for a manufacturer of running shoes. Commercial and market

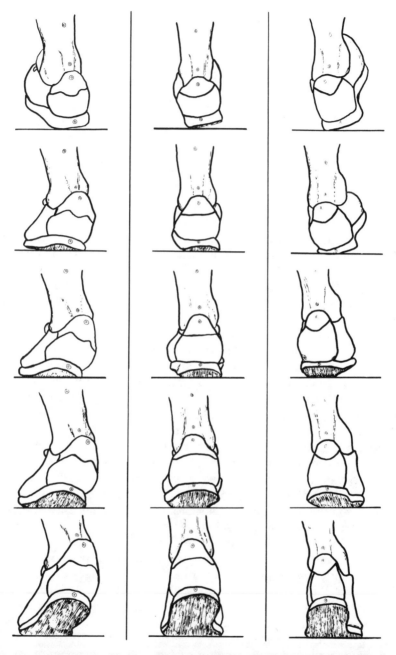

Figure 1.3. The rotatory position and movement in the ankle joint for three runners representing an overpronation (left), very little pronation (center), and also very little pronation but always remaining on the outside of the foot (right). All examples are of the left foot for heel-strike on the top and for intervals of about 50 m/s from top to bottom.

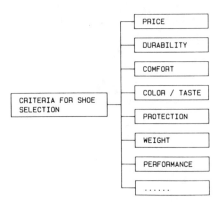

Figure 1.4. List of possible criteria for the selection of a running shoe.

analysis aspects may be included, together with technical considerations, and the importance of the various factors may differ in comparison to the runner.

However, the fact still remains that two out of three runners suffer an injury once a year, and there is no doubt that *protection against overloading* must be a very important aspect for everybody involved in running. Injuries in running are a consequence of overloading. Therefore, if we want to understand the origin of these injuries, we must study the factors influencing load in running, and how these factors can be influenced by the running shoe. The subjective judgment of cushioning of shoe sole material, for instance, may lead to wrong conclusions. If a runner examines a shoe by compressing the midsole with his or her fingers, he or she may find a shoe very soft. However, when using this shoe for running, the impact forces in the subtalar and ankle joint may be much higher compared to another shoe which may have appeared as being hard in a finger test. It may be that the feeling of the fingers is not in agreement with the feelings of the feet, joints, ligaments, and so on. It may be that a shoe sole is too hard and does not provide enough shock absorption, but it also may be that a shoe sole is too soft and bottoms out on every step. In order to protect runners from overloading, it has to be understood what overloading really means and where the origin of pain and injuries lies. If Cavanagh's statement that ''the percentage of runners getting injured did not change appreciably'' between 1973 and 1977 (Cavanagh, 1980) is correct, this could indicate that the development of sport shoe construction did not go in the right direction during this period of time. Therefore, it makes sense to systematically analyze the factors influencing loading of the locomotor system with the main emphasis on running shoes.

Protection against overloading must be one of the most important aspects in the construction and selection of a running shoe. However, there are many aspects which were or still are not completely understood in the relationship between running shoe construction, adaptation of the movement to a shoe, and load in the locomotor system. This book will concentrate on this relationship. It is assumed and will be illustrated that the construction of a running shoe is one important factor in reducing load in the body of a runner.

Loading of the Human Body

GENERAL COMMENTS

The human body is comprised of bone, cartilage, collagenous tissues (ligaments, tendon, and skin), soft tissue, and muscle. Each of these elements has different functions. *Bone* protects internal organs, provides rigid links and attachment sites for muscles, and facilitates muscle action and, therefore, body movement. *Cartilage*, covering the articular surfaces of bones, provides the functional connections between the different bones; this allows movement with minimum friction and spreads the loads over a large area, thus reducing local contact stresses. The prime function of *ligaments* is to stabilize the joint against extraneous motion outside of the normal dynamics of movement, to guide the joint motion, and to prevent excessive motion. The function of *tendon* is to attach muscle to bone and to transmit tensile loads. *Soft tissue* has the function of absorbing and distributing load. While all of these elements are passive, the *muscles* are active elements. Their function is to produce motion as well as to stabilize the internal locomotor system. All these body elements or body materials are constructed and adapted to carry load in one way or another.

The concept of load on the locomotor system is not always uniformly used (Nigg & Denoth, 1980). Therefore, the key term and its application is defined and explained.

Load is defined as the external forces which act upon a body.

This general definition which is analogous to load definition used in conventional material mechanics is explained and subsequently illustrated with three examples. The "body" upon which forces act can be anything—a piece of steel, a car, a bridge, and so on. However, in this book the "body" is the whole human body or parts of it. These parts can be an arm, a leg, a foot, or even more detailed, a bone, a piece of cartilage, or a tendon. Depending on the body of interest, the external forces may be forces outside the human body (if the whole human body is considered as a unit), or inside the human body (if an element is considered as a unit). Some examples may illustrate this.

1. Load on the human body in running are body weight, the forces due to air resistance, and the reaction force on the foot during floor contact. These forces are the only external forces acting on the human body. (Should the fellow runner next to you hit you at the start of a marathon, additional external forces would have to be considered!)
2. Load on the femur would consist of joint forces in the knee and hip joint, of forces at the attachment sites of tendons, ligaments, joint capsule, and of the weight of the femur.
3. Load on the Achilles tendon would consist of forces at the insertion of the tendon on the calcaneus, of forces due to friction of the tendon with the soft tissue, of forces at the attachment between tendon and muscle, and of the weight of the tendon.

Thus, load on the locomotor system is an important consideration of the construction and selection of a running shoe; therefore it is logical to discuss the factors which influence load in the locomotor system. A systematic subdivision is presented in Figure 1.5. The factors influencing load and stress in the locomotor system during running can be subdivided into two groups: the dynamic factors and the boundary conditions. The dynamic factors include type of movement (running, sprinting, jumping), the velocity of the center of mass (CM), the changes of body posture and muscular activity, and the number of repetitions

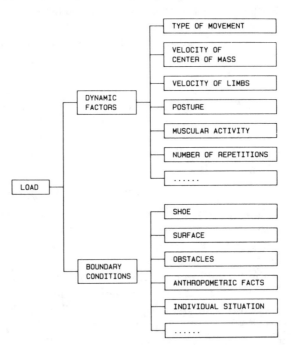

Figure 1.5. Schematic description of factors influencing load on the human body during running activities.

(steps per unit time). These dynamic factors can be influenced by the athlete. An athlete can change his or her running style from heel-toe to toe running or change his or landing velocity. In doing so, he or she can influence the load.

The boundary conditions include shoe, surface (e.g., grass or asphalt), obstacles (e.g., bumpy roads or uneven grass), anthropometric facts (e.g., leg length, mass distribution, varus or valgus position), and individual situation (fitness level). The athlete is able to change some boundary conditions in changing the shoes, running on grass instead of asphalt, or improving his or her fitness level. However, in many cases, the possible changes are limited. In some areas it is difficult to find grass for jogging, and anthropometric facts can usually not be changed. The only influencing factor in this list which can easily be changed is the shoe. Therefore, the following chapters concentrate on the shoe factor in order to understand how the running shoe can influence load on the locomotor system.

An analysis of load on the human body has two important aspects which have to be discussed in more detail. One aspect is the geometry of the acting forces which includes the point of application and the direction. A force acting at the forefoot may produce other internal forces in the Achilles tendon than if the same force were acting at the calcaneus. The second aspect is the loading rate which indicates how fast the acting force changes. The various structures in the human body may react differently to high-loading rates compared to low ones.

GEOMETRY OF ACTING FORCES

Depending on direction and point of application, external forces can produce tension, compression, bending, shear, and torsion. Tension is produced if equal and opposite forces are applied outward from the surface. The result is tensile stress in the inside, and the body reacts by changing its length and circumference (longer and more narrow). Structures in the human body which often experience this form of stress are tendons, ligaments, and muscles. Compression is produced if equal and opposite forces are applied to a structure toward the surface. The result is compressive stress in the inside, and the body reacts by becoming shorter and wider. Structures in the human body which often experience this form of stress are bone, cartilage, and some soft tissue. Bending results in a combination of tensile and compressive stress as illustrated in Figure 1.6 (Pauwels, 1973). This example underlines the importance of the geometry aspect: Two external forces of the same magnitude produce totally different results in the inside of a structure.

Bending usually occurs in rigid bodies. Bending stress can be observed in bone. Shear is produced by forces applied parallel to the surface of the structure. The result inside the structure is shear stress. Articular car-

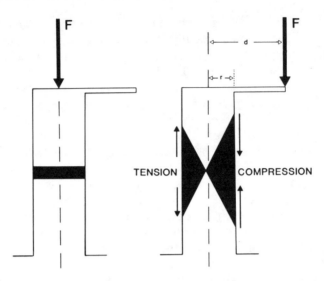

Figure 1.6. Schematic illustration of the effect of bending in an idealized structure.

tilage as well as soft tissues experience shear stresses. Torsion is produced by forces acting perpendicular and eccentric to an axis. The results are shear stresses distributed over the entire structure.

Living structures are very seldom loaded in only one way. Bone, tendon, ligament, and cartilage, for example, are constantly subjected to a sum of different stresses. This suggests that the analysis of stress on a living structure is extremely difficult. It may be possible to quantify with sufficient accuracy reaction forces on the ground during running. However, the determination of stress in internal structures may be much more complicated and sometimes even impossible. These explanations also show that the geometry of the human body is very important if one wants to study load on the locomotor system during an activity such as jogging. A person with a valgus leg may have totally different forces acting in the lateral collateral ligaments of the knee joint than a person with a varus position of the leg. A study of the factors influencing load on the human body without the consideration of the geometry is, therefore, inappropriate as it neglects one very important aspect.

LOADING RATE OF GROUND REACTION FORCES

Example 1. A person is standing on a force platform moving the trunk up and down. The related force time diagram in Figure 1.7 shows a relatively slow oscillation with body weight (BW) as the mean line. Because the test subject did not leave the force platform during the test, all the movements were produced by gravitation and by changes in muscular activity and were actively controlled by the muscular system. In this example, the maximal loading rate is about 9 N/ms (ms = milliseconds).

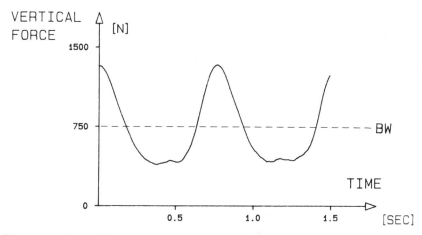

Figure 1.7. Vertical force-time curve for rhythmical up-and-down movement.

Example 2. Using the same time scale as in Example 1, the impact force of an iron shot dropping onto a force platform with a rubber cover 1 cm thick is illustrated in Figure 1.8. The force-time diagram for this laboratory experiment with a mass of 10 kg and an impact velocity of 4 m/s shows a brief signal with duration of about 40 ms. This experiment is an example of a typical impact phenomenon with an average loading rate of about 100 N/ms.

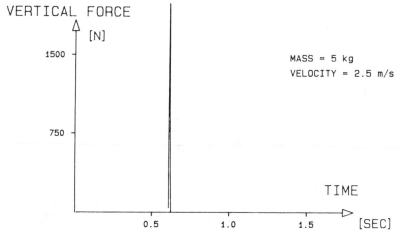

Figure 1.8. Vertical force-time diagram for a shot dropped onto a rubber cover (m = 10 kg and v = 4 m/s).

Example 3. A subject is running over a force platform. An accelerometer is mounted on the tibia. The foot contact in this example begins at the heel and ends at the toe (heel-toe running). The corresponding vertical force-time as well as the acceleration-time diagram for one foot contact are shown in Figure 1.9. The first part of the acceleration curve in direction of the axis of the tibia shows a shape similar to the result in Figure 1.8 (impact test), a signal with a duration of about 30 ms. The vertical force-time curve shows both types of shapes discussed in Examples 1 and 2, one with a relatively high-loading rate of about 150 N/ms at the begin-

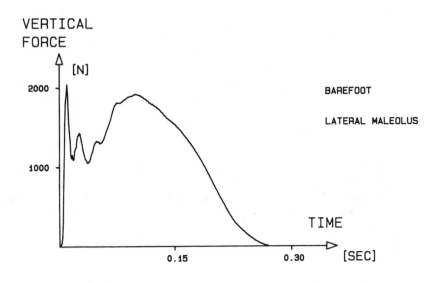

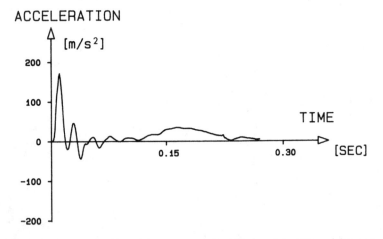

Figure 1.9. Vertical force and axial acceleration at the tibia as a function of the time for one foot contact in heel-toe running.

ning, and one with a slower loading rate of about 25 N/ms following this first peak. It could, therefore, be described as a superposition of two curves, one similar to Figure 1.8 and another similar to a part of Figure 1.7. Generally speaking, many force curves from human movement have two parts: a part with a high-loading rate, and a part with a low-loading rate. The frequency of the high-loading first part is about 10 to 15 Hz when using a sinusoidal description. The frequency of the second part with the lower loading rate is about 1-3 Hz. In order to distinguish these two parts, a value of 5 Hz seems to be appropriate, which corresponds to the description of impact in a mechanical sense.

In order to understand the significance of these two types of forces here is another example.

Example 4. An athlete performs a jump of about 3 meters over an obstacle of 30 cm. The movement after the take-off is about the same for all jumps and does not change during the experiment. The variable changing during the experiment is the approach velocity (2.5 m/s, 3.5 m/s, 4.5 m/s, 5.5 m/s, and 6.5 m/s). The result of the vertical and anterior-posterior (a-p) force-time function during take-off is illustrated in Figure 1.10. It shows force-time functions with a *low* and a *high frequency* part. The low frequency part looks pretty similar for the four different approach velocities. However, the high frequency part is relatively small for the slow approach velocity and relatively high for the fast approach velocity. The illustrated examples suggest that the high-frequency part is strongly correlated to the movement before ground contact. Furthermore, this example suggests that each movement has a typical vertical force-time curve (e.g., walking, running).

A camel type force-time curve for the vertical component is, for example, typical for walking; a parabolic type of the vertical force-time curve is typical for running. Because the movement after take-off in Figure 1.10 is always the same (a 3 m long and 30 cm high jump), the shape of the low-frequency part (vertical component) of all the five jumps is more or less identical.

The high-frequency forces are a result of an impact. The deceleration depends on the velocity of contact, the involved mass, the stiffness, the damping characteristics, and other factors. Because the approach velocity in Figure 1.10 is increasing, it may be assumed that the velocity of contact is increasing as well. This may be the reason for the increasing amplitude of the high-frequency force parts in Figure 1.10. Evidence for the correctness of this explanation can be shown with another experiment.

Example 5. A human leg is simplified as a rigid construction with one hinge joint. The lower leg (*tibia*) is represented by a mass m (m = 0.55 kg). The thigh is represented by a mass double that of the lower leg. The muscles are simulated by linear springs: One spring represents the knee flexors, another spring represents the extensors of the knee joint. This

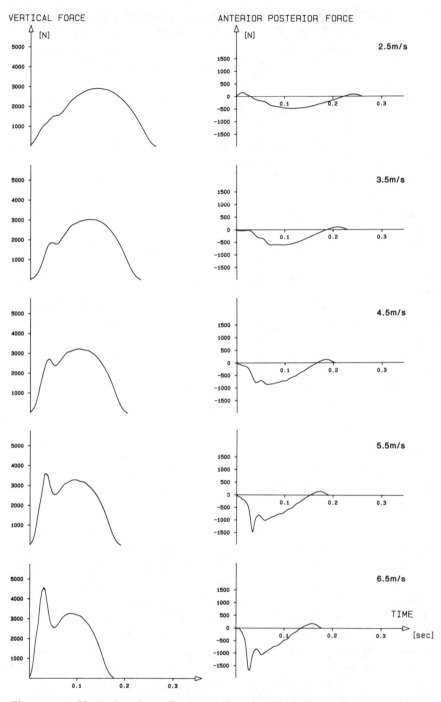

Figure 1.10. Vertical and a-p force-time function for a jump (3 m) with different approach velocities (in analogy to Kunz, 1978).

model is dropped on a force platform from different heights (10 cm, 20 cm, and 30 cm) with different knee angles (90°, 135°, and 180°) and different tensile forces of the springs. In order to simulate the human ability to adapt to different surfaces, the stiffness of the springs was varied (1.5, 8.5, 20, 40 N/cm). The tensile forces as well as the stiffness reported are for the spring at the anterior side of the knee joint representing the extensor muscle groups. The maximum impact forces resulting from these experiments are illustrated in Figure 1.11 (left side).

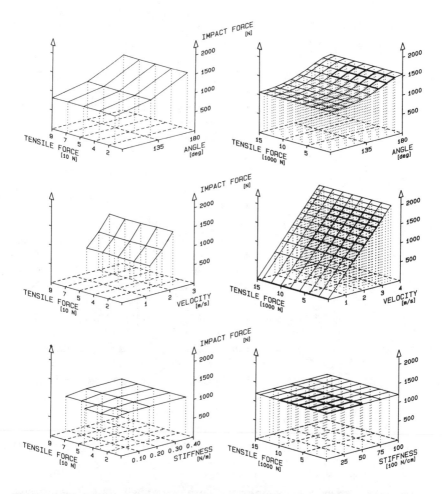

Figure 1.11. Average of the maximum impact forces as a result of the drop tests. Left-side experiment, right-side calculation. Top: velocity = 2 m/s, stiffness 40 N/cm; middle: knee angle = 135°, stiffness 40 N/cm; bottom: velocity = 2 m/s, knee angle = 135°. The thicker lines indicate results for the physiological range.

The measured range of stiffness does not correspond to stiffness values reported by Cavagna (1970) for subjects bouncing with locked knees (380 N/cm), Green and McMahon (1979) for subjects standing on both feet with knee angles of 45° (378 N/cm), and McMahon and Green (1979) during fast human running (sprinting) (730-1170 N/cm). However, other sources indicate that the stiffness of the leg for heel-toe running (3 m/s) on the treadmill is between 90 and 100 N/cm (unpublished values from Gordon Valiant of the NIKE Sports Research Laboratory). Because the experimentally determined impact peaks are measured with too low stiffness and tensile force values, a theoretical model was calculated using the same data for the two masses but increasing the tensile forces up to 15,000 N and the stiffness values up to 10,000 N/cm (unpublished results from A. Bahlsen, Calgary). These ranges include the physiological range which is indicated in the picture (Figure 1.11, right) with thicker lines. The results of the experiment and the model correspond well. They indicate that stiffness and tensile forces of the springs do not influence the magnitude of the impact forces in the physiological range, but that the knee angle at touch down and the velocity of touch down are very important. The maximal impact forces increase with increasing velocity. (For further information, see chapter 3).

Based on the five examples of this chapter, it seems meaningful to subdivide the force curves into a high frequency and a low frequency component. For this book, the high frequency forces which are connected with the first touch down of the contact element (e.g., heel) with the ground are called *impact forces* following publications by Frederick, Hagy, & Mann (1981), Clarke et al. (1983), and Nigg (1983). These impact forces in heel-toe running have their maximum at about 10-20 ms for barefoot running and at about 15-35 ms for running with running shoes (Cavanagh & Lafortune, 1980; Clarke et al., 1983; Nigg, 1983). The amplitudes of these vertical impact forces in heel-toe running can go up to 2 to 4 times body weight (BW) depending on running velocity, surface, and individual style. Impact forces for toe running are much smaller (less than body weight) and the peaks are reached earlier (5-15 m/s after first contact). The low frequency part of the force-time function will be called *active forces* (Nigg, 1980). It is the part of the force typically connected with the movement (running, walking, etc.).

The subdivision in impact and active forces (see Table 1.2) may include some sources for misinterpretation. The fact that one force aspect is called active may imply that the muscular system is activated in this interval. However, it may also suggest that it is not activated during the duration of the impact forces. Such an interpretation would be wrong. The muscles are turned on long before first contact (preactivation). There is, of course, tensile stress in the extensors of the knee, for example. Otherwise, the leg would collapse. This mechanical set-up is not able to react with a

Table 1.2. Specifications for impact and active forces (times in milliseconds = ms).

Force	Name	Frequency (Hz)	Time to maximum (ms)
High frequency	Impact	> 5	< 50
Low frequency	Active	< 5	> 50

change in activity in the relatively short-time interval of 15-35 m/s (Schmidtbleicher, 1980). However, the muscular activity changes in a feedback mode during the active phase of the force curve. The expression *active* refers therefore to the change in activity due to the nervous system to effect a specific movement. There are other ways to characterize the various phases of ground contact (Komi, 1983). However, for this book the words *impact* and *active* were chosen.

ORDER OF MAGNITUDE OF ACTIVE AND IMPACT FORCES

Active and impact forces have two independent origins. It is of interest to know the magnitude of the external and internal active and impact forces as well as some possible effects of these forces. External forces in the following examples are ground reaction forces acting on the human body. Internal forces are forces inside the human body.

External active forces in various activities have been measured by several authors. Naturally, most of the results describe walking. The results show that the maximal vertical active force is in the average about 1.2 times body weight, the maximum in a-p direction about 0.2 times body weight, and the maximum in mediolateral direction about 0.05 times body weight (Baumann & Stucke, 1980). The maximal vertical active force is the same for walking barefoot or in sportshoes. However, subjects with Achilles tendon pain show slightly higher maximal vertical forces (Nigg et al., 1984). The knowledge with respect to the active ground reaction forces in walking is very extensive because such measurements were performed for more than 100 years. Measurements of active ground reaction forces in running started later. The maximal active vertical forces in running are about 2.5 times body weight and the peak values in the two horizontal components are about 0.4 to 0.5 times body weight (Cavagna & Margaria, 1964; Cavanagh & Lafortune, 1980). Once again, there is no difference in the active vertical peaks between running barefoot and with running shoes (Nigg et al., 1984). The maximal active forces in sprinting are about 3.6 times body weight for the vertical, 0.8 BW for the a-p, and 0.4 BW for the mediolateral component (Baumann & Stucke, 1980). In general, we can summarize for the active forces that the vertical peaks double from walking to running and triple from walking to sprinting. The a-p component doubles from walking to running and quadruples from walking to sprinting. However, the mediolateral component remains quite constant.

Normally, *internal active forces* cannot be measured, but they can be estimated with the help of a model of the human body or parts of it. Possible forms of modelling, their limitations and problems, as well as their advantages are discussed in chapter 3. Some results of such estimations are presented in Table 1.4. However, it has to be mentioned that the shoe as a possible influencing factor has not yet been included in studies.

Internal active joint reaction forces in the hip joint in a dynamic situation were studied by Paul (1965, 1967), Seireg and Arvikar (1975), and other investigators. The results of their estimations showed maximal active hip-joint reaction forces slightly higher than 5 times body weight for men and about 20% less for women. For walking, the highest active forces in the hip joint are usually during take-off. However, the joint reaction force is not zero during swing phase because of the activity of the muscles holding together the joint. The resultant joint reaction force is always depending on effects of the external ground reaction force and effects of the muscle forces which are responsible for the agonistic and antagonistic activity. Dynamic (active) forces in the knee joint were estimated by Paul (1967), Morrison (1969, 1970), Seireg and Arvikar (1975), and others. The maximal joint reaction forces for walking were between 3 and 8 times body weight (see Table 1.3). Dynamic forces in the ankle joint were estimated by Seireg and Arvikar (1975). The maximal forces were 5.2 times body weight in walking. Baumann and Stucke (1980) estimated the ankle joint reaction forces for sprinting (13 times body weight). Procter and co-workers (1981) estimated the internal active forces in the subtalar joint during walking as 4 times body weight. Dynamic forces during walking in various muscle groups around the knee joint were estimated by Morrison (1970).

The maximal active forces were 2.3 times body weight for the hamstrings, 1.2 times body weight for the quadriceps femoris, and 1.5 times body weight for the gastrocnemius. This illustrates that the internal forces can easily be a multiple of the externally measured ground reaction forces. The active internal forces in normal walking are, therefore, 3 to 7 times body weight in the various joints of the lower extremities. They may even be greater in faster movements such as running and jogging. The corresponding active forces in the other elements of the locomotor system (muscles, tendons, ligaments, etc.) may easily reach multiples of body weight for activities such as running. Depending on the direction of the acting forces and the geometry of locomotor system, the stress pattern of specific elements can vary considerably. In jogging (toe landing), for instance, the stress of the anterior lateral cortex at toe-strike is primarily compressive (about 300 N/cm^2). It is followed by a high-tensile stress

Table 1.3. Estimated active internal forces in various types of movements for normal subjects with no specific footwear. The values with an asterisk (*) are calculated under the assumption of an average body mass of 70 kg.

Movement	Subject	Site	F_{max} (N)	F_{max} (BW)	Author	Year
Walking	Normal	Ankle joint	—	5.2	Seireg	75
Walking	Normal	Subtalar joint	—	4.0	Procter	81
Walking	Normal	Knee joint	—	4.6	Paul	67
Walking	Normal	Knee joint	—	4.0	Morrison	69
Walking	Normal	Knee joint	—	3.2	Morrison	70
Walking	Normal	Knee joint	—	7.1	Seireg	75
Walking	Normal	Hip joint	—	5.8	Paul	65
Walking	Normal	Hip joint	—	5.4	Seireg	75
Walking	Normal	Hip joint	3500	5.0*	Crowninshield	81
Walking	Normal	Spine L3-L4	—	1.8	Cappozzo	82
Walking	Impaired	Spine L3-L4	—	3.0	Cappozzo	82
Walking	Normal	Hamstrings	—	2.3	Morrison	70
Walking	Normal	Quadr. femoris	—	1.2	Morrison	70
Walking	Normal	Gastrocnemius	—	1.5	Morrison	70
Sprinting	Normal	Ankle joint	8900	12.7*	Baumann	80

Table 1.4. External vertical impact forces (ground reaction) in various types of movements. The values with an asterisk (*) are calculated under the assumption of an average body mass of 70 kg.

Movement	Velocity (m/s)	Footwear	F_{max} (N)	F_{max} (BW)	Author	Year
Walking heel-toe	1.3	Barefoot	—	0.6	Cavanagh	81
Walking heel-toe	1.3	Casual shoes	—	0.3	Cavanagh	81
Running heel-toe	2.7	Running shoe	—	2.8	Clarke	82
Running heel-toe	3.4	Barefoot	1365	2.0	Frederick	81
Running heel-toe	3.8	Barefoot	1590	2.3	Frederick	81
Running heel-toe	4.5	Running shoe	—	2.2	Cavanagh	80
Running heel-toe	4.5	Barefoot	1963	2.9	Frederick	81
Running heel-toe	5.5	Running shoe	2350	3.6*	Nigg	81
Running jump	6.0	Spikes	4000	5.3	Nigg	78
Running jump	8.0	Spikes	5500	7.9*	Nigg	81

(about 1100 N/cm²) during push off (Lanyon, 1975). This result is due to the different bending of the tibia.

Measurements and calculations of external and internal active forces have been performed for decades. Measurements of external impact forces have only been performed for a few years, and impact forces have only recently been used in connection with running shoe analysis. The external impact force peaks in the vertical direction in running (see Table 1.4) are between 2 and 4 times body weight for running or jogging with heel-toe contact (Nigg et al., 1978, 1981; Cavanagh & Lafortune, 1980; Frederick et al., 1981; Clarke, Frederick, & Cooper, 1982). They are dependent on the type of movement, the velocity of touch down, the shoe, and the surface as well as the involved mass which will be demonstrated later. These are factors that can be influenced by the athletes and the sport equipment manufacturers and are, therefore, of great interest in this book. They will be discussed in depth in chapters 3 and 5. We are convinced that the understanding of this aspect is the key to further improvement of running shoe construction.

External impact forces can also be estimated in connection with acceleration measurements at the tibia or other locations of the human body. Therefore, some of the measurements published earlier may be relevant for considerations in connection with external (as well as internal) impact forces if the boundary conditions are known.

Methods for the calculation or estimation of *internal impact forces* were developed by Nigg & Denoth (1980) and used mainly in connection with playing surfaces. Results using these methods (see Table 1.5) show joint reaction forces in the ankle joint of about 0.4 times body weight in walking, 1 to 6 times body weight in running (heel-toe), and up to more than 10 times body weight in other landing movements. The joint reaction forces in these landing movements in the knee joint are up to 8 times body weight.

The results of measured and estimated forces in the lower extremities in walking, running, and jumping show that active as well as impact forces

Table 1.5. Summary of estimated maximal internal impact forces in various types of movements.

Movement	Velocity (m/s)	Location	F_{max} (N)	F_{max} (BW)	Surface	Author	Year
Walking	0.4	Ankle	300	0.4	Grass	Denoth	81
Walking	0.4	Ankle	300	0.4	Synth	Denoth	81
Running heel-toe	0.8	Ankle	700	1.0	Grass	Denoth	81
Running heel-toe	0.8	Ankle	1200	1.7	Synth	Denoth	81
Running heel-toe	1.5	Ankle	1300	1.9	Grass	Denoth	81
Running heel-toe	1.5	Ankle	3700	5.3	Synth	Denoth	81
Running heel-toe	—	Ankle	1600	2.3	Synth	Nigg	80
Running heel-toe	—	Knee	1100	1.6	Synth	Nigg	80
Landing	5.5	Ankle	1800	2.6	Synth	Nigg	80
Landing	5.5	Knee	900	1.3	Synth	Nigg	80
Landing gym	9.0	Ankle	7200	10.3	2 Mats	Nigg	80
Landing gym	9.0	Knee	5900	8.4	2 Mats	Nigg	80

in elements of the human body can easily be a multiple of body weight. Impact forces can be greater as well as smaller than active forces. They are usually smaller than the active ones for slow movements (such as walking) and can be greater than the active forces in fast (e.g., fast-heel running or take-off for jumping), as illustrated in Figure 1.10.

SIGNIFICANCE OF ACTIVE AND IMPACT FORCES

Little detailed knowledge is available, and in many cases, there is not even agreement on most of the general questions. This section is an attempt to develop a general system which describes various aspects of the effect of forces and stresses on biological materials.

Mechanical stress on biomaterials has two effects:

1. A short-term effect where the material reacts in a mechanical way. Examples for such reactions are bending or torsion.
2. A long-term effect where the material shows responses of a living structure. Examples include increasing cross-sectional areas of muscles, tendons change in the chemical structure, or alignment of internal bone structure (Pauwels, 1973).

The measurement of external forces is, as illustrated, well under control. The tools are available and the quantification of these forces has been performed quite frequently. The estimation of internal forces is already more complex and connected with several problems. However, the understanding of the biological effects of forces acting on the locomotor system is very difficult and still needs further development.

Mechanical deformation of dead material has critical limits. The material is damaged if these limits are exceeded (fractures, microtraumas, tears, etc.). If the stresses are kept below these critical limits, then the resulting deformations are usually only present as long as the mechanical stress is acting. The material will immediately, or after a relatively short time (hysteresis), get back to its original form. On the other hand, a stimulus in the form of stress is necessary for the development of biomaterials such as bone, cartilage, tendon, ligament, or muscles. No force or too little force (too little stimulus) causes bionegative effects which can easily be demonstrated with immobilized parts of the locomotor system. Muscles, tendons, and so on quickly change (degenerate) their mechanical properties. A plastercast for 4 weeks, for example, on the lower leg and foot reduces the critical limits of the involved structures drastically (Butler, Grood, Noyes, & Zernicke, 1978). Excessive forces cause bionegative effects which can be chronic or acute. A fracture, for instance, may be the result of a single force which produces a stress well beyond critical limits. As another possibility, it may be a result of a repeated application of relatively normal forces. Such fractures then are called *fatigue fractures* and depend mainly on the frequency of repetitions, the amplitude of the forces, and the critical limits.

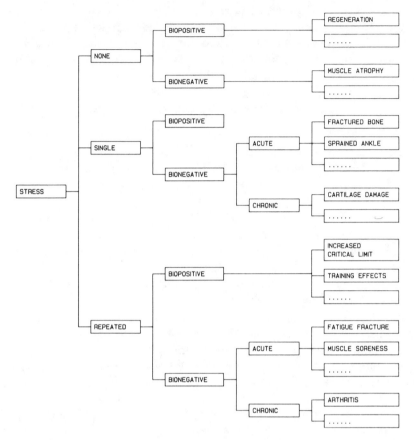

Figure 1.12. A proposed systematic analysis of the effect of forces acting on the human body.

Figure 1.12 is an attempt to systematically understand the connection between the various possibilities of effects produced by different applications of force. It shows that forces and stresses on biological materials can have biopositive or bionegative effects. Bionegative, however, is not only a possible result of overloading but can be a result of too little load (see Figure 1.13). A *medium load* band width exists where, for a given frequency of repetition, the effect on specific material is positive.

These biopositive or bionegative effects as illustrated in Figure 1.13 depend on the subjects as well as on many other factors, one of them being the type of force. We speculate that impact forces are critical for the etiology of pain and injuries in many sports activities (Nigg et al., 1974), and that they are connected with the occurrence of chronic injuries (Nigg, 1983). This speculation is supported by other authors. Radin and co-workers (1973) could show that degenerative changes in cartilage can rapidly be produced by impact forces of relatively large amplitude. Light and co-workers (1980) speculate that impact force transients play a role in the development of osteoarthritic changes. They add that these impact forces may be connected with back troubles and fatigue failures and even act as triggering agents in neurological diseases. Voloshin and Wosk (1982) report that the body's capacity to attenuate acceleration to the spine caused by impact forces is about 20% worse in subjects with low back pain compared with normal subjects, and they conclude that these results suggest a plausible theory for the explanation of low back pain. Radin and co-workers (1982) have shown that biochemical and mechanical characteristics of knee cartilage of sheep changed when they walked on concrete compared to another group walking on compliant wood chips. The experiment does not allow a final conclusion as to whether these changes would eventually lead to true osteoarthrosis over a prolonged period of time. However, some similarity to questions like cushioning and shoe or surface cannot be denied.

Results by Falsetti, Burke, Feld, Frederick, & Ratering (1983) indicate that increased red blood cell destruction is related to mechanical trauma (impact forces) in running and may be influenced by the cushioning characteristics of the sole of a running shoe. All these examples of studies support the general speculation that impact forces (especially in heel-toe running) may have a bionegative effect. The fact that about two out of three runners are afflicted with running injuries during the period of a year indicates that obviously the forces and stresses acting on the locomotor system are too high for the repetition rate used. For many runners or joggers, the load in Figure 1.13 would be on the right side and the effects are obviously bionegative.

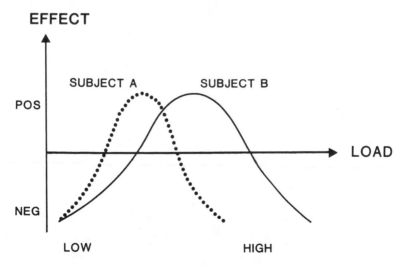

Figure 1.13. Schematic representation of the effect of forces and stresses on the human body (Nigg & Denoth, 1980).

2

BENNO M. NIGG

Experimental techniques used in running shoe research

Various approaches can be used to study a special field such as biomechanical aspects of running shoes. The problems can be studied using theoretical (analytical) techniques using mathematical models and some of these are discussed in chapter 3. Another common technique is the *experimental* (empirical) approach using measuring systems which seem to be appropriate in answering the questions connected with the field of interest. Historically, the experimental approach usually precedes the theoretical approach. This was also the case in the field of running shoes. Various measuring systems were adapted or developed, and the sophistication of these systems in the field of running shoe analysis is probably more advanced than the few theoretical approaches reported in the literature. This does not at all imply that the experimental approach is more powerful than the theoretical one. It suggests that the experimental approach is often used to "get the feeling" for the movements, forces, and torques involved in running because this knowledge was not available.

Chapters 2 and 3 are designed to describe the techniques used for both the experimental and the theoretical approaches. Because these two approaches are in two different chapters does not imply that in reality they should be separated. A meaningful research strategy would include both techniques because both have their strengths. Chapter 2 describes the experimental techniques used in running shoe analysis and includes the quantification of kinematic and kinetic variables (movement and forces) as well as the assessment of material properties such as the elements of the shoe and the surface.

Measurement of Force and Moment

The main external forces acting on the human body during running are ground reaction forces acting on the runner during contact with the ground. These forces can be measured with a measuring device called *force platform*. The platforms commonly used are based on piezo electric or strain gauge techniques and have resonance frequencies usually above 300 Hz. The force platforms allow the quantification of the ground reaction force F and its components F_x, F_y, F_z, the point of application k and its components k_x and k_y and the free moment of rotation around the vertical axis M_z with respect to the point of application.

The force is a vector and we use the following convention for the direction of the three components:

F_z = *Vertical force*
Definition: Component of ground reaction force in vertical direction. Comment: F_z is always positive which means that the positive z-direction is upward.

F_y = *Anterior posterior (a-p) force*
Definition: Component of ground reaction force in a-p direction. Comment: F_y is positive in the running direction. The initial a-p ground reaction force in running is therefore negative and the final a-p ground reaction force is positive. They describe the braking and the propulsive phases (see Figure 2.1).

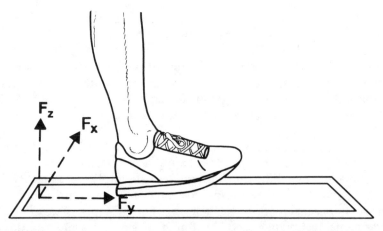

Figure 2.1. The direction of the components of the ground reaction forces.

F_x = *Medio-lateral force*

>Definition: Component of the ground reaction force in medial or lateral direction, perpendicular to the running velocity.
>
>Comment: F_x is defined as positive to the medial side of the athlete looking in running direction. F_x is therefore usually negative at the beginning of ground contact and mostly positive during stance phase.

This convention will be used consistently throughout the book. Other publications may use symbols and conventions in a different way. This system has the advantage to compare results from left and right feet immediately. However, it is not a right turning system of coordinates. If vector calculations are used, this must be taken into consideration.

Figure 2.2 illustrates an example of the three force-time components. The left side of the graph shows mean and standard deviation for 10 trials

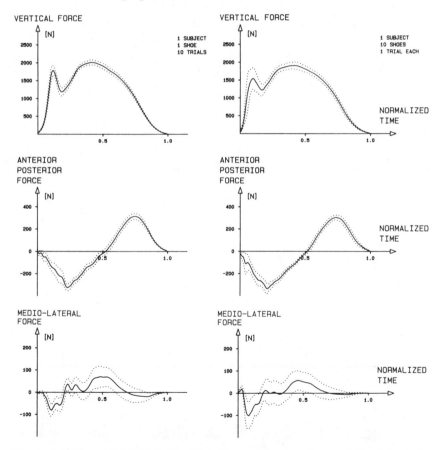

Figure 2.2. The reliability (left) of 1 subject with one shoe and 10 trials and the variability (right) of the same subject and 10 different shoes for heel-toe running (3.5 ± 0.2 m/s).

for 1 subject running with the same speed. It illustrates, therefore, the reliability of these force measurements. The right side shows an average for 10 trials for the same subject. However, these measurements were made with 10 different shoes. It illustrates, therefore, the variability of force measurements with different running shoes. One may expect that the variation of the force curves for 1 subject with constant boundary conditions are clearly smaller than the variation for 1 subject running with 10 different running shoes used in this experiment. The result shows that this is only correct for the early sections in the graph (impact peaks). The shoe obviously plays a dominant role in this respect, and it is evident that this variable is sensitive in the description of running shoes. The most common variables used for analysis of the force-time function are listed in Table 2.1.

The list of possible variables can be easily expanded. However, this list summarizes the variables commonly used for the force analysis. As mentioned in Table 2.1, impact force peaks are not always visible. This is illustrated in Figure 2.3 which shows the vertical force time averages for 1 subject running 10 trials with Shoe 1 (a running shoe) and 10 trials with Shoe 2 (a tennis shoe). It is obvious that in this example, Shoe 1 shows a very clear impact peak while Shoe 2 does *not* show an impact peak. The magnitude of the impact peak is obviously shoe dependent. There are, of course, other factors which influence the impact peaks (Luethi, 1983; Nigg, 1983).

Another variable to describe the load during impact is the maximal loading rate. We assume that this variable has a physiological significance because it is connected with stretching velocities of human tissue. Furthermore, this variable has the advantage to exist in every force curve

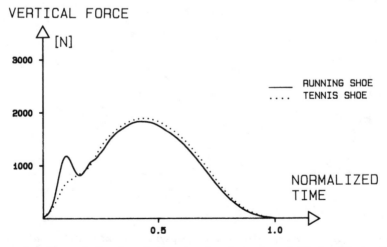

Figure 2.3. Example for the occurrence of an impact peak for 1 subject with 10 trials each for two different shoes (mean curves).

Table 2.1. Variables used in the force-time analysis.

Symbol	Name	Explanation
T	Contact time	Duration of ground contact
F_{zi}	Vertical impact force peak	Maximum of the vertical impact force in the first 50 m/s
F_{yi}	a-p impact force peak	Maximum of the a-p impact force corresponding to the vertical impact peak
F_{xi}	Medio-lateral impact force peak	Maximum of the lateral impact force corresponding to the vertical impact peak (Note: The impact peaks may not be visible in one or several components.)
t_i	Time of impact peak	Time interval between the first ground contact and the occurrence of impact peak
G_{zi}	Maximal vertical loading rate	= grad $(F_z)_{max}$ — maximal time derivative (loading rate) in the vertical direction before the impact peak (maximal slope)
G_{yi}	Maximal a-p loading rate	Ditto for a-p direction
G_{xi}	Maximal medio-lateral loading rate	Ditto for medio-lateral direction
t_{zG}	Time of maximal vertical impact slope	Time interval between the first ground contact and the occurrence of the maximal vertical impact slope
t_{yG}	Time of maximal a-p impact slope	Ditto for a-p direction
t_{xG}	Time of maximal medio-lateral impact slope	Ditto for medio-lateral direction
F_{za}	Vertical active force peak	Maximum of the vertical active force (after the impact peak)
F_{ya+}	a-p active force peak (accelerating)	Maximum of the a-p active force during take-off (positive)
F_{ya-}	a-p active force peak (decelerating)	Maximum of the a-p active force during the first half of ground contact (decelerating)
F_{xa+}	Medio-lateral active force peak (inward)	Maximum of the medio-lateral active force in inward direction
F_{xa-}	Medio-lateral active force peak (outward)	Maximum of the medio-lateral active force in outward direction
I	Integral	Area under the force-time curve (Note: There are various possibilities to define the integrals (absolute real, relative to BW).

while the impact peak is sometimes not visible. The relationship between these two variables is illustrated in Figure 2.4. The values are from 1 subject running at four different velocities (3, 4, 5, and 6 ± 0.2 m/s) with three different shoes. The result may suggest a quadratic relation.

There is obviously a variation in this relationship when including more subjects as illustrated in Figure 2.5. It shows the correlation between the impact force peak F_{zi} and the maximal loading rate G_{zi} for 16 subjects wear-

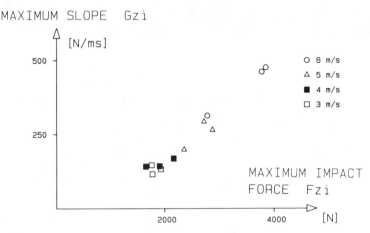

Figure 2.4. Relationship between the impact force peak F_{zi} and the maximal loading rate G_{zi} for 1 subject running with three different shoes at four different velocities (3, 4, 5, and 6 ± 0.2 m/s).

ing the same shoe for four different running velocities. However, the result supports the findings for 1 subject illustrated in Figure 2.4

It is obvious that the force-time curves depend on the velocity of running as illustrated in Figure 2.6. It shows the force-time curves for the same four running velocities with 16 subjects all wearing the same shoe. The curves show that the vertical and lateral impact peaks increase with increasing velocity. The contact time decreases. The active force maxima change very little in the vertical direction but significantly in the a-p direction due to the required propulsion. The pattern of the lateral force seems

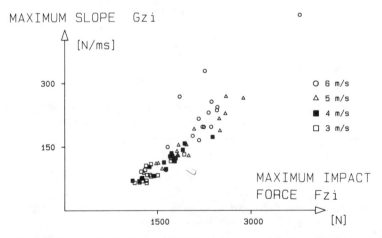

Figure 2.5. Relationship between the impact force peak F_{zi} and the maximal loading rate G_{zi} for 16 subjects running at four different velocities (3, 4, 5, and 6 ± 0.2 ms) with three different shoes.

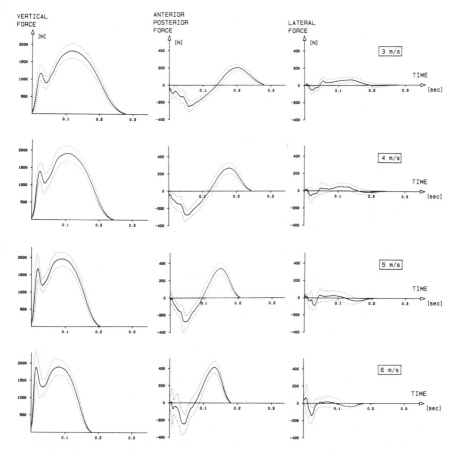

Figure 2.6. Average force-time curves with standard deviation for four running velocities (3, 4, 5, and 6 ± 0.2 m/s), 16 subjects, and one shoe. The curves are normalized with respect to the corresponding average contact time. Note that for the highest speed the subjects are still accelerating.

to change systematically. These illustrated changes underline that information from force-time curves is only meaningful if the running velocity is known (Frederick et al., 1981).

The *point of application* in the horizontal plane is the point on the force platform from where the force vector starts $P(k_x/k_y)$. This point is quite clearly an application point when a rope is fixed to a car. It is also an application point in the example illustrated in Figure 2.7 where a heel of a running shoe touches the ground at first contact.

However, when the whole shoe sole is in contact with the ground, it may be confusing to speak about a point because forces are acting all over the shoe sole. Therefore, it is appropriate to call this point *center of pressure* as used by Cavanagh and Lafortune (1980).

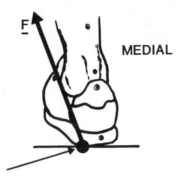

Figure 2.7. Point of application (center of pressure) in heel-toe running.

k_y = *a-p coordinate of center of pressure*
Definition: Location of the origin of the ground reaction force in y-direction.
Comment: k_y has usually a system of coordinates which is connected with the force platform. The positive and negative values do not have a special meaning and are arbitrary. However, we use the convention that the movement of the subject is in the direction toward the positive y-axis.

k_x = *Medio-lateral coordinate of center of pressure*
Definition: Location of the origin of the ground reaction force in x-direction.
Comment: k_x is defined as being positive toward the lateral and negative toward the medial side.

The center of pressure can be illustrated in various ways. One possibility is the drawing of the center of pressure as a function of time as illustrated in Figure 2.8 for the a-p direction. The first vertical line on the time axis indicates the moment of first contact with the ground; the second one indicates the last contact. Due to accuracy problems, the center of pressure cannot be determined for small vertical forces. The first point in the curve which can be used is B (begin) which is a few milliseconds after first contact and the last point is E (end) which, again, is before the last contact. The straight line BE signifies a rolling with constant velocity from one point to another point on the force platform. The curved line between B and E is the path of center of pressure for a selected subject. In this example, the subject lands on the heel ($k_y = -13$ cm), and the center of pressure moves relatively fast to the midfoot of the sole. The take-off is at about $+10$ cm (point E). The variables commonly used for analysis are listed in Table 2.2.

Other forms of illustration were published by Stuessi, Aebersold, and Debrunner (1978) and Cavanagh and Lafortune (1980) and are presented in Figure 2.9. The 3-D illustrations are very instructive in showing the location of the center of pressure in combination with the magnitude and

CENTER OF PRESSURE IN A-P DIRECTION ky

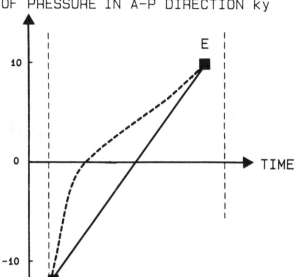

Figure 2.8. Center of pressure as a function of time for the a-p direction. Example of 1 subject running with running shoes at a velocity of 3 m/s and a stride length of 1 m.

direction of the force vector for equal time intervals. The illustration by Cavanagh and Lafortune (left side) even includes the position of the shoe during contact allowing a comprehensive view of a total ground contact. The two methods are suitable for fast analysis and may be used successfully in clinical and/or diagnostic situations. The quantification in connection with k_x, k_y, and the time as illustrated in Figure 2.8 has the advantage that variables can be calculated and used for quantitative comparison; therefore, it will have more use in research.

The *free moment* about an axis parallel to the z-axis through the center of pressure $P(k_x/k_y)$ has the symbol M_z. This moment is produced by the runner, and it is normal that moments exist during ground contact.

Table 2.2. Variables used for the analysis of the center of pressure-time function.

Symbol	Name	Explanation
k_{xmax}		Maximal distance between the center of pressure-time curve and BE, parallel to the k_x axis
k_{ymax}		Ditto for k_y
I_{BE}	Integral	Area between the line BE and the center of pressure-time function (x and y)

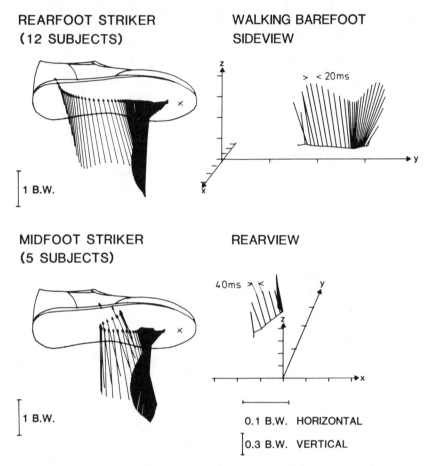

Figure 2.9. Graphic display of center of pressure and force vectors by Cavanagh and Lafortune (left) for running and Stuessi et al. (right) for walking. Reprinted by permission.

M_z = *Free moment of rotation*

  Definition: Moment of rotation with respect to a vertical axis through the center of pressure.

  Comment: In analogy to the convention in the force measurements, we study the answer of the force platform. A moment which resists an outward rotation is defined as a *positive moment*.

Using this convention, the moments during running are usually *positive* (resisting outward rotation) at the beginning of ground contact and *negative* (resisting inward rotation) at the end of foot contact. Factors which influence these moments are the friction between shoe and surface and the geometrical construction of the human body.

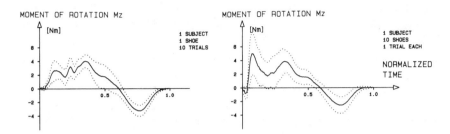

Figure 2.10. Normalized moments about the vertical axis for running heel-toe with a slow velocity of 3 m/s (mean and SD). Left: 1 subject, 1 shoe, 10 trials. Right: 1 subject, 10 shoes, 1 trial each shoe.

Figure 2.10 shows moment-time curves (mean and SD) for 1 subject running 10 times at 3.5 m/s heel-toe with one shoe, and the same subject with the same velocity but running in 10 different running shoes (same experiment as in Figure 2.2). The graph shows that the standard deviation for different shoes is generally about the double of the standard deviation for one shoe which suggests that this variable is sensitive to changes in shoes. A comparison with the corresponding values of the force measurements shows that the variability of the moments (standard deviation divided by the mean) is about 5 to 10 times bigger. This illustrates that it is much more difficult to detect differences in shoes with moment measurements than with force measurements. The variables commonly used in moment measurements are listed in Table 2.3

A review of the research performed with force platforms in the field of running shoe studies reveals that most of it is done by using the vertical force-time function. There is very little published work using horizontal forces, center of pressure, or moment of rotation. The few publications which use the latter variables are mostly methodological in describing techniques or indicating ranges and mean values (Cavanagh, 1978a, b;

Table 2.3. Variables used for the analysis of moments about the vertical axis through the center of pressure.

Symbol	Name	Explanation
M_{max}	Maximum moment	Maximum value of M_z resisting outward rotation
M_{min}	Minimum moment	Maximum value of M_z resisting inward rotation
G_m	Maximal rotational loading rate	Grad $(M_z)_{max}$
I	Integral	

Cavanagh & Lafortune, 1980; Williams, 1982). One of the few exceptions is Winter (1984) who showed that the within-subject variability of kinematics and ground reaction forces is quite low, but the variability of moments is much higher. He concluded that moments are a very sensitive tool for gait analysis, producing important basic knowledge. However, there were no other researchers who used these techniques and the connected variables in applied running shoe analysis. The reason for it is not evident. It may be due to the fact that the variability of vertical forces is much smaller, or that the vertical forces are considered to be more relevant because they are much bigger than the horizontal ones.

Measurement of Pressure Distribution

A very comprehensive description of the kinetics during ground contact is the measurement of pressure distribution. Instead of measuring one resultant reaction force, a system of unidirectional force transducers is used with areas as small as .3 cm × .3 cm. It is evident that an immense sum of information is contained in a pressure distribution display, and it is a logical consequence that various techniques were developed with increasing interest in gait and running. The earliest pressure distribution measurement goes back to Abramson in 1927. Later, Elftman (1934) used a system with rubber pyramids in contact with a glass plate and a film camera. This idea was later used by Miura and co-workers (1974). Arcan, Brull, & Simkin (1976) quantified pressure distribution with light interference methods. Nicol and Hennig (1976) used a flexible mat as a capacitor and 256 capacitor plates on each side. The advantage of such a system is that only 32 channels are required on each side of the pressure distribution device.

Clarke (1980) used such a system to collect pressure distribution data for 27 subjects. An example of these measurements is illustrated in Figure 2.11a and 2.11b for walking. It is obvious that a very large amount of information is portrayed in these pictures. Cavanagh and Michiyoshi (1980) used a device similar to Arcan and quantified pressure distribution beneath the foot in slow walking. A new pressure distribution measuring technique was developed by Lord (1981) and the group of the Penn State Biomechanics Laboratory (Cavanagh et al., 1983; Hennig, Bunch, & Macmillan, 1983). It is a device designed as an insole in this example with 499 elements of about 5 mm square based on piezoelectric principles. It was the first time that the pressure distribution between foot and shoe could be shown with such a high resolution.

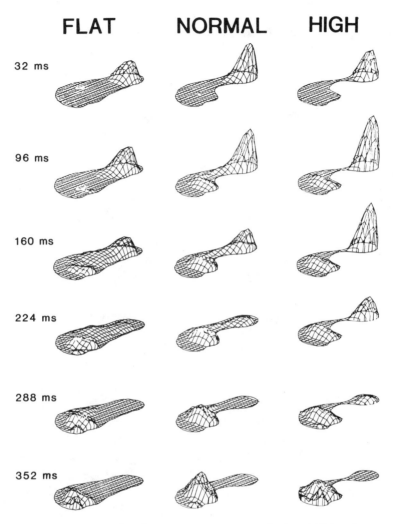

FLAT **NORMAL** **HIGH**

32 ms

96 ms

160 ms

224 ms

288 ms

352 ms

Figure 2.11a. Pressure distribution measurements during walking from Clarke (1980). Reprinted with permission.

Another approach in pressure distribution quantification is the use of pressure-detecting sheets (Aritomi, Morita, & Yonemoto, 1983). There is no doubt that a large number of methods are available. However, these methods were not widely used for running shoe analysis. To my knowledge, only one research laboratory (Penn State) has applied this technology for running shoe analysis. An example of such a display is illustrated in Figure 2.11b (from Cavanagh).

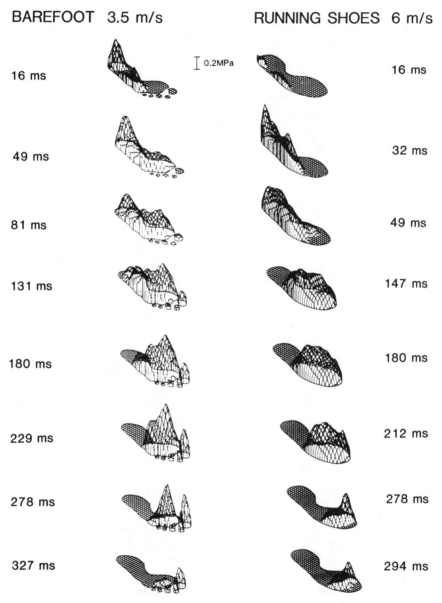

Figure 2.11b. Pressure distribution measurements during running from Cavanagh. Reprinted with permission.

Measurement of Movement

Many measuring techniques are used in connection with research in running shoes. However, optical methods are most frequently used, for they allow the quantification of kinematic variables such as angle, change in angle, position, displacement, and velocity. The various techniques used are conventional film systems, video-based systems, and systems using LEDs (light emitting diodes). In addition to these "classical" techniques that cover the vast majority of studies performed in connection with running shoes, other optical methods can be applied (chronozyclography, impulse photography, etc.). All of these methods involve some sort of a picture which contains the information of the location of a number of markers and the time. The analysis of this information is identical for all these systems. For this reason, only *film and film analysis* will now be discussed. The comments and results can easily be adapted to the other optical systems.

In an attempt to quantify the influence of running shoes on the kinematics of the lower extremities, in 1975 we filmed subjects with different running shoes from posterior, medial, lateral, and anterior views. The results of this pilot project showed differences in kinematic variables for different shoes for the posterior and lateral views. These two filming directions were then used in the following years and are still in use in our laboratories as well as in other centers of research with running shoes. These methods will be discussed later. A comprehensive summary of the analysis of rearfoot movement based on kinematic variables from the posterior view has been published by Clarke et al. (1984). The description in this chapter will not repeat this overview but will describe in detail the method developed by our group (Nigg & Luethi, 1980).

The rear view of one foot contact of a heel-toe runner usually shows a landing on the ouside of the rear part of the foot followed by a *rolling inward* of the foot, usually in the first 50% of contact, and a *rolling outward* during take-off. The first part, called *pronation*, is a complex motion consisting of simultaneous eversion, abduction, and dorsiflexion. The second part, called *supination*, is the reverse movement (inversion, adduction, and plantar flexion). Every optical method describing this complex movement is connected with problems. The most critical problem is that usually markers on the skin (relative movement of skin with respect to the skeleton) and on the shoe (relative movement of shoe with respect to the skeleton) are used. Based on the results of various studies, the markers on the rear part of the leg, heel, and heel cap, respectively, are placed as illustrated in Figure 2.12.

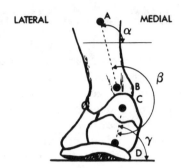

Figure 2.12. Illustration of the markers at the rear part of a left leg and foot.

A   Located 15 cm above marker B in the center of the leg (rear view) in the standing position (barefoot)
B   Located on the Achilles tendon just above the heel cap of the shoe
C   Located on the upper part of the heel cap
C   Located so that the line between CD and the horizontal form an angle of 90° in the unloaded shoe
D   Located in the center of the shoe sole (posterior view)

If a subject is running barefoot, the markers C and D are located on the heel of the subject so that they form an angle of 90° with the horizontal in the static standing position on two legs. Using the projection of these markers into the x-z plane, the following angles can be defined:

α = *Angle of the lower leg*
   Definition: Angle between AB and the horizontal line on the medial side.
   Comment: The angle of the lower leg contains information about the kinematics of the lower leg (tibia). It is specific for subjects and running style.

β = *Achilles tendon angle*
   Definition: Angle between AB and CD on the medial side.
   Comment: The Achilles tendon angle contains information about the relative angular movement between calcaneus and lower leg. It is therefore used to describe pronation and supination.

γ = *Rearfoot angle*
   Definition: Angle between CD and the horizontal line on the medial side.
   Comment: The rearfoot angle contains information about the shoe. The time history of the Achilles tendon angle and the rear foot may be different.

It is obvious that these three angles are redundant. The connection is

$$\alpha + 180° = \beta + \gamma$$

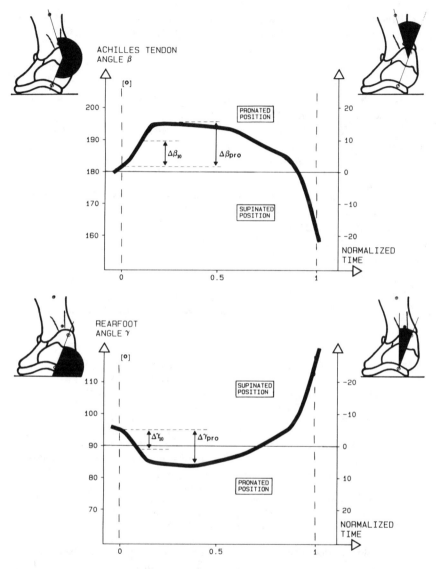

Figure 2.13. Angle of the Achilles tendon angle and rearfoot angle during ground contact in heel-toe running for 1 subject with 4 m/s.

Therefore, knowing two of the angles allows the calculation of the third. In some cases, it may be useful to use all three angles. An example of the time history of these angles during ground contact is illustrated in Figure 2.13. The left axes indicate the variables as defined earlier. The right axes illustrate similar variables used by other groups. No basic difference exists between the two solutions.

In this example, the subject lands with a rearfoot angle of about 95° and an Achilles tendon angle of about 182°. The subject pronates and has a maximal pronated position at 0.16 of the total foot contact and the maximal pronation position of the heel at 0.39 of the total foot contact time. The example illustrates that the Achilles tendon and rearfoot angle may have their maximum or minimum with a phase shift. The variables used in connection with the rear view film analysis are defined and explained in Table 2.4. The convention consistently used in this context is that angular positions at a defined time are labeled with a Greek symbol, α, β, or γ, and that relative changes in angles are labeled with $\Delta\alpha$, $\Delta\beta$, or $\Delta\gamma$.

The list of variables can easily be expanded. Various researchers have used the listed, similar, or even additional variables (Bates et al., 1978; Bates et al., 1979; Clarke et al., 1984; Clark et al., in press). The variables listed in Table 2.4 can be grouped in the following way:

Table 2.4. Variables used in the kinematic analysis (posterior view).

Symbol	Name	Comments
β_o	Initial Achilles tendon angle	Achilles tendon angle immediately before first ground contact
β_{pro}	Maximal Achilles tendon angle	Measured at the time of maximum pronation
$\Delta\beta_{10}$	Initial pronation	Change of the Achilles tendon angle in the first 10th of foot contact
$\Delta\beta_{pro}$	Total pronation	Total change of the Achilles tendon angle during the pronation part of foot contact
$\dot{\beta}_{10}$	Initial pronation velocity	Average angular velocity of β during first 10th of foot contact
$G(\beta)_{max}$	Maximal pronation rate of Achilles tendon angle	$\dot{\beta}_{max}$ = maximal value of the angular velocity of the Achilles tendon angle
β_{end}	Take-off angle Achilles tendon	Achilles tendon angle 1/10 before last foot contact
γ_o	Initial rearfoot angle	Rearfoot angle immediately before first ground contact
γ_{pro}	Minimum rearfoot angle	Measured at time of maximum pronation
$\Delta\gamma_{10}$	Initial change of rearfoot angle	Change of the rearfoot angle during the first 10th of foot contact
$\Delta\gamma_{pro}$	Total pronation of rearfoot angle	Total change of the rearfoot angle during the pronation part of foot contact
$\dot{\gamma}_{10}$	Initial rearfoot velocity	Average angular velocity of γ during first 10th of foot contact
$G(\gamma)_{max}$	Maximal pronation rate of rearfoot angle	γ_{max} = maximal value of the angular velocity of the rearfoot angle

Initial conditions:	β_o	γ_o
Initial changes:	$\Delta\beta_{10}$	$\Delta\gamma_{10}$
	$\dot{\beta}_{10}$	$\dot{\gamma}_{10}$
	G_β	G_γ
Maximal pronation:	$\Delta\beta_{pro}$	$\Delta\gamma_{pro}$
	β_{pro}	γ_{pro}
Take-off:	β_{end}	

The variables describing an angular position are more dependent on the positioning of the markers than the variables describing a change in an angle. Figure 2.14 shows an example of the time history of the three angles for 1 subject running with one shoe, mean and standard deviation for 10 trials on the left, and running with 10 shoes with one trial for each shoe on the right side. Figure 2.14 illustrates the reliability and variability for 1 subject. It indicates that the initial conditions are not as sensitive to shoe changes as the variables describing pronation and supination during ground contact. Note that in this example, the running shoes represented a selection of high quality shoes with similar construction. It is expected that the result noted above would show greater variation if the whole range of running shoes was analyzed.

There will always be a discussion to what degree the markers on the shoe represent the markers on the skin of the heel and/or the position of the calcaneus. The first aspect (shoe-heel) was studied with a project where holes in the heel cap allowed observation of both markers (Figure 2.15). The results of measurements with one shoe, 3 subjects, and three trials per subject and shoe showed a systematic shift of 2-3° between the two rearfoot angle curves. However, the shape of the curve is the same and the differences between the heel and shoe variables describing a change are smaller than 1°. It may be that the agreement is reduced in extreme cases (e.g., pronatory movement in the Achilles tendon angle of more than 30°).

Another factor which is important are the initial conditions. They are crucial for the (impact) reaction forces, the movement of the lower extremities and the rest of the body. A change of the touch down velocity of the heel from 0.8 m/s to 1.4 m/s as indicated later can have a significant influence on the impact forces and on the subsequent pronation. The initial conditions which are important are

- touch down velocity
- area of contact at touch down
- geometry of the contacting leg

for a given subject/surface combination. These variables can be quantified or estimated by using film pictures from the lateral view (in connection with posterior view). Figure 2.16 illustrates the markers used for the filming from the lateral side. The markers are located as follows:

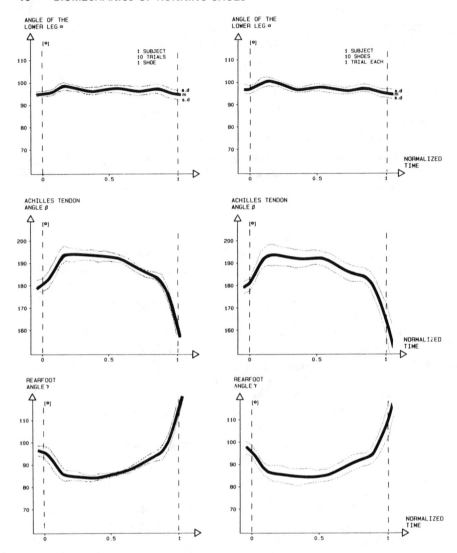

Figure 2.14. Example of the angle of the lower leg, the Achilles tendon angle, and the rearfoot angle during ground contact (v = 3.5 m/s). Left: 1 subject, 1 shoe, 10 trials. Right: 1 subject, 10 shoes, 1 trial each.

E   Midsole of forefoot at the head of the 5th metatarsal
F   Midsole of the heel underneath the calcaneus
G   Lateral maleolus
H   Head of the fibula
I   Located above the knee joint (tibio-femoral joint on a middle line for lateral view in the standing position)
K   Same as I but ⅔ of the distance between the tibio-femoral and the hip joint

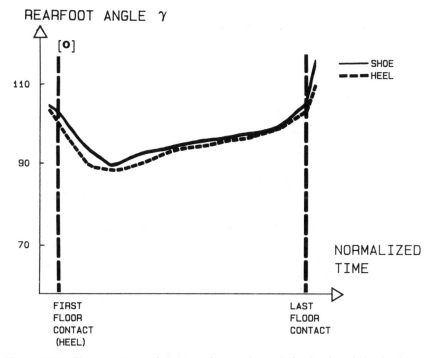

Figure 2.15. The agreement between the markers at the heel and the heel cap of the shoe (one shoe, 3 subjects, three trials per subject and shoe). From unpublished results of Stacoff, Zurich.

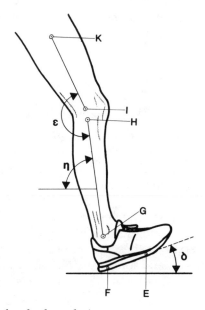

Figure 2.16. Markers for the lateral view.

Using these markers, the following variables can be defined, all of them being angles and velocities projected into the y-z plane:

ϵ = *Knee angle*
Definition: Angle betwen GH and IK on the posterior side of the knee joint.
Comment: This angle is important for the determination of the effective mass and internal impact forces (see chapter 3).

δ = *Angle of the shoe sole*
Definition: Angle between EF and the ground measured at the lateral side.
Comment: This angle is connected with the area of contact and the lever arm of the acting force with respect to a specific joint.

η = *Angle of the lower leg* (lateral)
Definition: Angle between GH and the horizontal line at the posterior side.
Comment: This angle is important for the calculation of internal forces during ground contact.

v = *Velocity of the heel*
Definition: Velocity of the lateral maleolus (point G) before and during contact.
Comment: This velocity usually is subdivided into two components, a vertical and an a-p component. The vertical component is important for the vertical impact forces.

One frequent use of thee variables is the determination of the initial conditions. They are defined as the values of these variables immediately before first ground contact and are consistently labeled with an index o (ϵ_o, δ_o, η_o, v_o, and, of course, α_o, β_o, γ_o).

Material Tests and Tests With Subjects

Tests with test subjects are usually associated with problems of reliability and are very time consuming. This encourages the use of material tests which are not affected by these problems. Mainly three groups were involved in the development of material tests in connection with running shoes: SATRA, the Footwear Technology Centre in England, the Biomechanics Laboratory of The Pennsylvania State University, and the American Society for Testing and Materials FO8.54 Subcommittee on Athletic Footwear. Some of these test procedures were, and are, used internally by companies, and some were used for assessment of running shoes for practical use (Cavanagh, 1978). There is agreement that such tests must be valid if they are applied for advising buyers of running shoes. This means that knowledge on the material properties as well as

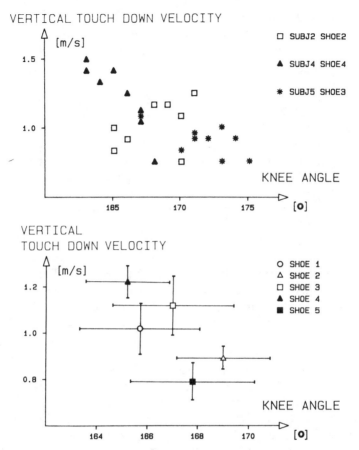

Figure 2.17. Knee angle and vertical touch down velocity. Top: 3 subjects, eight trials with different running velocities, each subject with one special shoe. Bottom: mean values for 5 subjects (left and right foot) for five different shoes (running velocity 3.5 m/s).

on the movement is necessary. In order to understand this comment, the connection between the shoe and the vertical touch down velocity is illustrated in Figure 2.17. The subjects were instructed to perform heel-toe running. The results show ranges in the average knee angles immediately before first contact of 3.8° and for the vertical touch down velocity of 0.43 m/s. These results show that touch down velocity is especially sensitive on shoe construction.

Another experiment with 1 test subject using 15 different shoes during treadmill running showed that the initial angle of the lower leg α_o varied between 92° and 97°, and that the initial rearfoot angle γ_o varied between 97° and 105°. These results illustrate that the shoe obviously influences the movement pattern and that these changes can be quite significant, greatly influencing the impact forces (most likely not taken into account in material tests). This example contains other information. The bottom part of Figure 2.17 shows results that are connected with the shoe. The figure shows that the average population has a relatively low touch down velocity in running with Shoes 2 and 5 but has a much higher one for Shoes 3 and 4. This is a very interesting result but not the end of the story. The top part of Figure 2.17 gives more information with respect to individual runners. The result shows that each of the 3 subjects has an individual strategy in running with his or her own shoe. The result underlines that various aspects are important in analyzing impact forces in connection with running shoes, the material properties, the movement pattern, and the possible strategies of individual runners.

This first example describing problems of impact measurements with material tests is just one aspect of load analysis. Similar comments can be made for friction measurements. Frictional forces are of great importance for mobility of the human being in the horizontal plane. Without frictional forces, it would not be possible to accelerate or decelerate the human body. Pedestrians, for instance, have problems walking on an icy road due to lack of friction between shoe and ground. In the case of sport shoes, frictional forces are important from a performance point of view as well as from a medical point of view. High friction between shoe sole and floor is desired in order to increase the reaction of an athlete (fast deceleration and acceleration). On the other hand, the friction should be decreased so that the maximum load, acting on the body, is below the critical physiological limit in order to prevent pain and injuries (Segesser, 1976). To judge different types of running shoes according to their frictional behavior, the frictional forces which may occur and the transition point between the physiological and nonphysiological load situations where only the question of the determination of the frictional forces is addressed must be known.

There are various possibilities for measuring translational friction coefficients (Bowers & Martin, 1975; Van Gheluwe, Deporte, & Hebbelinck, 1983; Perkins & Wilson, 1983; Schlaepfer et al., 1983). All of them use the horizontal and vertical forces in order to calculate the friction coefficient, which is a material constant. Coulomb friction can be used for friction measurements with running and tennis shoes and surfaces (Nigg & Denoth, 1980; Schlaepfer et al., 1983). Experiments for the quantification of friction coefficients were performed with five different surfaces. Surface #1 was artificial grass, #2, #3, and #4 were artificial surfaces, and #5 was an artificial surface with loose granulate (slide). Five different shoes were used in varying the material as well as the tread. The results are illustrated in Figure 2.18 showing a significant influence of the surfaces on the frictional behavior of the shoe soles. A difference of about 25% between the friction coefficient of Surface #1 (artificial grass) and Surface #4 (Porplastic SW) could be observed. An additional decrease of more

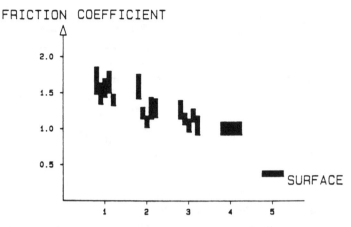

Figure 2.18. Range of friction coefficient for five sport shoes in connection with various surfaces.

than 30% could be achieved by using loose granulate on Surface #3. By comparing the differences of the frictional coefficients within the various shoes and within the various surfaces, it may be stated that within the used set of test shoes and surfaces, the influence of the surface on the friction coefficient is dominant. However, it is not clear if the structure or the material of the surfaces, or both, were responsible for the dominance.

The results for translational friction show that the expected range for static and dynamic friction coefficients is in the order of magnitude of about 0.3 to 2.0 for shoe-surface combinations. These results describe the frictional characteristics of several shoe-surface combinations. They are a typical material property. As in the previous example (impact), the human subject is included in the analysis in quantifying the resistance against rotation measured with the maximal moment of rotation. The experiment for the analysis of the rotational friction behavior was performed with 5 test subjects, seven shoes, and five surfaces. The shoes were the same as those used for the translational friction measurement. In addition, Shoe 1 and Shoe 2 were used. The surfaces were identical to the ones used for translational friction experiments. The test movement was a turn of 180° on the forefoot of one leg. The subject was allowed to hold onto a table with one hand during the test movement in order to provide a more reliable movement. The summary of the results for these rotational movements is presented in Table 2.5.

The average maximal moments of rotation for the surfaces used range from 10.6 to 20.1 Nm. From the resistance point of view, these surfaces probably represent a wide range. Another aspect is the variation of the shoes. The average values range from 12.8 to 17.9 Nm. In this case, it

Table 2.5. Average maximal moments of rotation for a 180° turn on one leg with different shoes and surfaces for 5 subjects.

Shoe	Surface 1	Surface 2	Surface 3	Surface 4	Surface 5	Mean
		Moment of rotation (Nm)				
1	13.2	12.8	14.9	13.5	9.5	12.8
2	20.1	16.2	18.7	23.8	10.5	17.9
6	18.6	14.7	17.1	20.4	10.4	16.2
7	18.1	15.6	17.5	20.8	11.1	14.6
8	17.9	14.7	16.9	21.1	11.2	14.4
9	18.2	14.6	16.7	21.7	10.5	16.3
10	17.5	14.8	16.9	19.1	10.9	15.8
Mean	17.7	14.8	17.0	20.1	10.6	

is assumed that the whole range of shoes currently available on the market is not represented. The conclusion of these results, therefore, would be that from the point of view of resistance against rotation, both the shoe and the surface may contribute significantly. The contribution of both can be of about the same order of magnitude.

Combining the material test with that of the test subjects, one may ideally expect that the two results are correlated. Figure 2.19 shows such

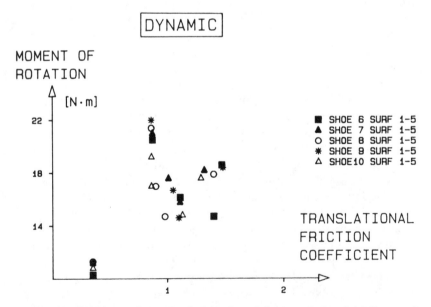

Figure 2.19. Correlation between the results of the translational friction coefficients and the maximal moments of rotation for 5 subjects, seven shoes, and five surfaces.

a combination between the dynamic friction coefficient and the moment of rotation. Obviously, it is not possible to use friction coefficients to determine moments of rotation without additional information. The result may be influenced by different construction properties of the shoes or different behavior of the subjects analogous to the impact results.

The two examples clearly illustrate the problems of using isolated material tests. Each shoe and special shoe construction influence the movement pattern of runners. Material tests, therefore, must include the effect of the shoe on the movement in order to be used as valid sources of information. However, this may be a very different undertaking.

General Comments on Measuring Techniques

No doubt there are other experimental techniques which could be used for the analysis of running shoes, for instance, measurements with accelerometers (Unold, 1974; Clarke et al., 1983). However, the main methods used are film and force analysis. This may be because of the availability of these methods in many laboratories, because of the information which can be gathered, or because of a combination of several reasons. However, the emphasis will be on results from studies with force and film analysis connected with experimental approaches. The two aspects discussed here in more detail are the sampling frequency and the selection of variables.

The *frequency* used for data sampling depends on the maximum frequency present in the studied movement. Procter (1980) and Marcus (1983) assumed that the maximum frequency present in walking is not higher than 10 Hz. Baumann and Procter (in press) state later that frequencies well in excess of 5 Hz can be found in gait. Based on the assumption of a maximum frequency present of 20 Hz, the sampling rate for walking would have to be set at least at 100 Hz using Shannon's sampling theories. The maximum frequency present in running is considered to be higher (Marcus, 1983). However, frequency spectrum analysis indicates that the maximum frequency present was never higher than 50 Hz. Therefore, the sampling frequency should be about 250 Hz. There are no problems in this context with force platform measurement because sampling rates are usually 1000 Hz or higher.

The film frequencies present a more severe hurdle because of costs and digitizing time. However, such frequency considerations are relevant if every aspect of a movement is studied. It may well be that the variables of interest are less frequency dependent. The maximum pronation position for the Achilles tendon angle, for instance, can easily be determined for running with a film frequency of about 100 frames/second. The variables listed in Table 2.4 are relatively insensitive with respect to frequency. Based on this, film frequencies between 100 and 200 Hz are considered to be sufficient for running.

Many aspects can be checked on in the *selection of the variables* to use for the study of running shoes. If there were only one or two variables available for analysis of running shoes, the following paragraphs would not be necessary. However, as Tables 2.1 to 2.4 show, many variables are available for use. We will discuss three aspects which may have some importance on the selection: a statistical aspect, a logical aspect, and an aspect describing the boundary conditions.

STATISTICAL ASPECTS

As a first step, one would not select a variable for which the intraindividual range is of the same order of magnitude as the range produced by the different shoes. This aspect is illustrated in Table 2.6 and contains some of the most frequently used film and force variables—the standard deviations. SD1 is the standard deviation for 1 subject, *one* shoe, and 10 trials with this shoe. SD10 is the standard deviation for 1 subject, *10* shoes (run-

Table 2.6. Standard deviation for film and force variables for 1 subject, *10* shoes, and one trial per shoe (SD10); and 1 subject, *one* shoe, and 10 trials with this shoe.

Variable	Unit	SD10	SD1	SD10:SD1
T	ms	14	10	1.4
γ_o	deg	2.6	2.7	1.0
γ_{pro}	deg	3.3	1.5	2.2
$t(\gamma_{pro})$	ms	21	23	0.9
$\Delta\gamma_{10}$	deg	2.9	1.8	1.6
$\Delta\gamma_{pro}$	deg	2.8	2.4	1.2
β_o	deg	2.7	3.0	0.9
β_{pro}	deg	4.4	3.1	1.4
$t(\beta_{pro})$	ms	32	28	1.1
$\Delta\beta_{10}$	deg	4.0	1.7	2.4
$\Delta\beta_{pro}$	deg	3.4	2.4	1.4
β_{end}	deg	5.5	3.1	1.8
α_o	deg	1.8	1.3	1.4
α_{pro}	deg	2.0	1.6	1.3
$t(\alpha_{pro})$	ms	11	54	0.2
F_{zi}	N	129	72	1.8
t_i	ms	38	6	6.3
G_{zi}	N/ms	54	14	3.9
t_{zG}	ms	4	1	4.0
F_{za}	N	94	71	1.3
F_{xa-}	N	54	25	2.2
F_{xa+}	N	32	49	0.7

ning shoes), and one trial for each shoe. The quotient SD10:SD1 can be used to decide whether a variable can be used with respect to variability. The results show that the listed force variables have generally high quotients (SD10:SD1). The vertical impact force peak (F_{zi}), its time of occurrence (t_i), the maximal loading rate (G_{zi}), its time of occurrence (t_{zG}), and the (initial) maximal outward force in lateral direction (F_{xa-}) all show quotients higher than 1.5.

The best variables for film analysis are the initial pronation values ($\Delta\gamma_{10}$ and $\Delta\beta_{10}$), the maximum pronation of the shoe (γ_{pro}), and the take-off angle (β_{end}). The times of occurrence of the maximal pronation is not shoe sensitive. There are, of course, limitations with respect to the results of this example, for they are only from 1 subject running at one speed. Some of the results could change if more subjects were included. However, results of previous measurements show that the general trend does not change. Based on this, the possible variables are as follows:

F_{zi}	Vertical impact force peak
t_i	Time of impact peak (vertical)
G_{zi}	Maximal vertical loading rate
t_{zG}	Time of G_{zi}
F_{xa-}	Lateral active force peak (outward)
$\Delta\gamma_{10}$	Initial change of rearfoot angle
$\Delta\beta_{10}$	Initial change of Achilles tendon angle
$\Delta\beta_{pro}$	Total pronation
γ_{pro}	Minimum rearfoot angle
β_{pro}	Maximum Achilles tendon angle
β_{end}	Take-off angle (Achilles tendon angle)

There are, of course, possible variables which are not included in Table 2.6. This table only contains variables commonly used in film and force analysis with running shoes. Some of the variables one may expect to be influenced by running shoes are not. The active vertical force peak, for instance, is *not* shoe sensitive; it is primarily movement sensitive.

LOGICAL ASPECTS

The main reason to select a variable for a study is, of course, not the variability aspect discussed in the previous pages: It must be a reason which is relevant for the operation under investigation. Two major aspects developed in the past years in running shoe research are performance, and load and injuries. If the interest is in performance, one can easily measure the running time (as a quantification of performance) and assess the influence of special shoe construction with respect to the final time. This procedure is affected by many disturbing side effects so that in research, usually the measurement of oxygen consumption is used. Various material characteristics in a shoe and construction strategies can be tested using this approach (Catline & Dressenhofer, 1979; Frederick et al., 1980; Clement et al., 1982; Frederick, 1983; Frederick et al., 1983; Hayes, Smith, & Sanpietro, 1983). Results of such studies show that performance can be influenced by shoe construction. The methodology in this context is basically clear, and hence there is no debate as to which variables are to be used. However, the situation changes when load and injuries are the topics of interest.

Ideally one should know the variables which describe the main factors causing injuries and pain. Because one does not have that knowledge, one must depend on speculation, supportive evidence, and medical experience. The solution to this problem is to find the connection between the cause and the result (pain). However, this has proved to be very difficult, has consumed many years of research to date, and is currently one of the most important topics in running shoe research. In the meantime, a temporary model based on the following three aspects is used:

- Landing impact
- Pronation
- Take-off supination

The landing impact (in this case we speak about heel landing) is considered to have a negative influence primarily on cartilage and bone (Radin et al., 1973; Light, McLellan, & Klenerman, 1980; Voloshin & Wosk, 1982; Radin et al., 1982). Falsetti (1983) supports the assumption that impact forces have bionegative effects with the finding of increased red blood cell destruction with increased impact force amplitude. It may be that there is also a connection to the shin splint problem. To summarize:

Impact forces: Damage: Cartilage
                          Bone
                          Shin splint
              Variables: F_{zi}
                         t_i
                         G_{zi}
                         t_{zG}

Pronation is a natural part of the foot movement during the support phase and is connected with rotation in the lower extremity, the ankle joint, the subtalar joint, and the transverse tarsal joint (Mann, 1982). The elements in the human foot limiting pronation are mainly passive structures (ligaments and bone contours). Furthermore, pronation in a dynamic sense (change of position) has to be optimal during ground contact in running. No pronation at all would mean a more rigid foot with less potential to absorb impact forces (d'Ambrosia & Douglas, 1982; Luethi, 1983).

Overpronation may strain supporting ligaments and connective tissue and is considered in the majority of cases as being the origin of pain and injuries. Lateral compression syndrome of the knee (Leach, 1982), illiotibial band syndrome (Leach, 1982), Achilles tendinitis and posterior tibial tendinitis (Clancey, 1982), and many other running injuries are assumed to be connected with overpronation. Some medical specialists working extensively with runners have the opinion that overpronation is one of the main causes of pain in most of the patients they treat (Segesser, 1970; Clement, 1982). Seemingly, overpronation is clinically relevant, and changes in sport shoe construction should usually reduce pronation. This statement is supported by the experimental finding that pronation in barefoot running is significantly smaller than in running with running shoes (see Figure 2.20, Nigg, 1983). To summarize:

Pronation: Damage: Ligaments
Soft tissue
Tendon insertion

Variables: γ_{pro}
β_{pro}
$\Delta\gamma_{10}$
$\Delta\beta_{10}$
$\Delta\gamma_{pro}$
$\Delta\beta_{pro}$

The third aspect in our model is oversupination during take-off. If a runner takes off on the outside of the forefoot and rotates the heel

ACHILLES TENDON ANGLE β

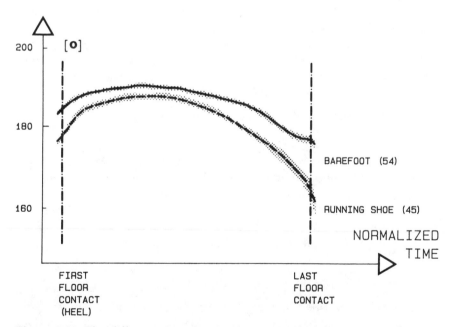

Figure 2.20. The difference in pronation in running barefoot (n = 54) and with running shoes (n = 45) with a velocity of 3 m/s (heel-toe running).

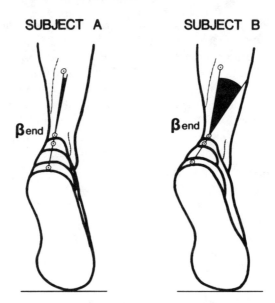

Figure 2.21. The take-off angle (Achilles tendon angle) for 2 different subjects. Note that methodological problems may occur due to the camera position (projected angle).

medially, the Achilles tendon angle may be as low as 160° (see Figure 2.21). However, the force in the Achilles tendon is maximal during take-off. One would, therefore, expect friction problems in the surrounding tissue at the medial side and/or stress problems in the lateral aspect of the Achilles tendon. Furthermore, it is assumed that excessive take-off angles are connected with high stress in the insertion of the tibialis anterior (Segesser et al., 1980). To summarize:

Take-off supination: Damage: Achilles tendon
                                      Insertion tibialis anterior
                Variables: β_{end}

It is assumed that the described variables are able to quantify factors which are connected with running injuries. Obviously, this aspect of research with running shoes needs some improvement.

However, by comparing the development of the empirical methodology with the development in the analytical theoretical approach, one can see that the empirical aspect is much more advanced than the latter one.

INITIAL AND BOUNDARY CONDITIONS

The variables described and used for running shoe studies most likely are sensitive to changing initial and boundary conditions. One boundary condition of interest in this context is the running velocity. Table 2.7 sum-

Table 2.7. Mean and standard deviation of variables used in the analysis for four different running velocities (± 0.2 m/s) and two different midsole hardnesses (shore A measurements). Details of the experiments are found in chapter 5.

Variable	Unit	Shore 25				Shore 45			
		3 m/s	4 m/s	5 m/s	6 m/s	3 m/s	4 m/s	5 m/s	6 m/s
γ_o	deg	99.8 (3.6)	99.6 (4.5)	101.9 (4.8)	101.9 (5.8)	99.8 (4.6)	100.1 (4.6)	100.7 (5.8)	101.6 (3.7)
γ_{pro}	deg	88.5 (2.8)	88.9 (3.0)	88.7 (3.6)	88.8 (3.2)	87.9 (1.7)	87.4 (2.3)	87.7 (2.0)	87.5 (2.4)
$t(\gamma_{pro})$	ms	125.0 (28.4)	109.0 (45.0)	67.3 (24.5)	69.0 (25.6)	137.2 (25.2)	104.9 (26.8)	80.0 (22.6)	65.2 (29.0)
$\Delta\gamma_{10}$	deg	2.0 (5.1)	1.2 (3.3)	2.6 (4.8)	3.0 (4.5)	5.8 (3.8)	4.7 (2.8)	4.4 (5.2)	5.3 (3.5)
$\Delta\gamma_{pro}$	deg	11.3 (5.4)	10.7 (4.3)	13.2 (6.0)	13.2 (4.4)	12.0 (5.2)	12.7 (4.0)	13.0 (6.1)	14.1 (3.3)
β_o	deg	179.8 (4.4)	179.3 (5.2)	178.3 (5.5)	179.0 (5.2)	178.9 (4.4)	179.0 (5.1)	179.2 (6.1)	179.9 (3.8)
β_{pro}	deg	193.6 (2.9)	193.4 (4.4)	195.7 (4.8)	197.4 (4.5)	194.0 (2.9)	195.2 (3.6)	197.3 (4.0)	199.0 (4.8)
$t(\beta_{pro})$	ms	136.3 (19.9)	101.9 (28.4)	81.6 (30.6)	82.7 (25.6)	134.4 (19.6)	117.1 (17.1)	88.2 (26.7)	70.6 (29.0)
$\Delta\beta_{10}$	deg	2.9 (5.7)	3.0 (3.5)	4.8 (5.2)	5.8 (5.0)	7.4 (4.3)	6.6 (3.2)	6.8 (5.3)	8.6 (4.7)
$\Delta\beta_{pro}$	deg	13.8 (6.1)	14.2 (5.1)	17.4 (6.6)	18.4 (4.3)	15.0 (5.8)	16.2 (4.2)	18.1 (6.4)	19.1 (4.5)
β_{end}	deg	168.8 (9.7)	167.6 (10.1)	167.6 (12.8)	164.2 (9.9)	168.8 (7.3)	169.5 (10.6)	167.4 (9.9)	168.3 (11.2)
α_o	deg	99.6 (2.9)	98.9 (2.7)	100.2 (2.5)	101.0 (4.1)	98.7 (2.0)	99.1 (2.3)	99.9 (2.5)	101.5 (3.4)

Table 2.7. (Cont.)

Variable	Unit	Shore 25				Shore 45			
		3 m/s	4 m/s	5 m/s	6 m/s	3 m/s	4 m/s	5 m/s	6 m/s
α_{pro}	deg	103.1 (3.1)	103.7 (3.6)	105.6 (3.4)	107.6 (4.3)	102.5 (2.7)	103.7 (3.2)	106.0 (3.8)	108.0 (5.0)
$t(\alpha_{pro})$	ms	119.3 (85.2)	90.1 (40.3)	100.0 (40.8)	84.1 (28.6)	106.4 (50.4)	109.8 (53.7)	90.2 (36.9)	81.5 (34.4)
F_{zi}	N	1373 (192)	1643 (311)	2014 (454)	2232 (477)	1302 (211)	1493 (229)	1798 (396)	2165 (416)
t_i	ms	30.2 (3.3)	25.1 (2.8)	23.5 (5.8)	17.9 (4.6)	25.2 (3.2)	23.3 (2.4)	19.1 (2.6)	16.5 (4.6)
G_{zi}	N/ms	87.7 (19.4)	115.0 (29.6)	162.8 (55.5)	221.8 (83.2)	96.3 (23.1)	115.5 (21.6)	157.0 (51.7)	240.8 (95.3)
t_{zG}	ms	18 (3)	15 (2)	13 (2)	10 (3)	14 (3)	12 (2)	10 (2)	7 (2)
F_{za}	N	1846 (172)	1952 (184)	2008 (216)	1943 (261)	1854 (203)	1927 (217)	1988 (196)	1925 (223)
F_{za-}	N	78 (41)	93 (47)	136 (47)	183 (91)	85 (31)	107 (32)	126 (47)	190 (80)
F_{za+}	N	69 (26)	81 (38)	63 (59)	74 (60)	87 (30)	88 (41)	86 (60)	70 (40)
v_{ez}	m/s	0.9 (0.3)	1.3 (0.4)	1.8 (0.8)	1.8 (0.4)	1.0 (0.4)	1.2 (0.4)	1.5 (0.5)	2.1 (0.6)
ϵ_o	deg	161.9 (4.5)	158.9 (5.0)	152.2 (8.4)	144.0 (7.2)	161.4 (3.7)	158.6 (5.9)	150.4 (7.4)	144.2 (8.7)
δ_o	deg	18.9 (5.0)	19.5 (7.1)	17.5 (6.6)	10.0 (9.4)	19.8 (4.7)	20.1 (7.0)	17.5 (6.0)	12.4 (8.8)

marizes the results of measurements with different running velocities (3, 4, 5, and 6 ± 0.2 m/s) for 16 subjects wearing a shoe with a relatively soft midsole (shore 25) and another shoe with a harder midsole (shore 45). The table shows that some of the variables are extremely velocity sensitive (impact force, loading rate, times of occurrence), some are sensitive in a smaller range but still significant (maximum pronation β_{pro}, γ_{pro}, $\Delta\beta_{pro}$), and some are not influenced by the running velocity. Therefore, it is crucial to control the running velocity if results should be compared for various shoes.

3

JACHEN DENOTH

Load on the locomotor system and modelling

Segments of the human body are constantly under mechanical stress whether a person is sitting in an armchair, standing, walking, running, or jumping. A certain amount of mechanical stress is necessary for the development of bone tissue, bone structure, muscle, and the nervous system. The determination or estimation of stress in a segment of the human body during a given activity is one aim of load analysis. The load distribution in the biological material in comparison to the load capacity allows us to quantify overload. This can be used to describe the quality of shoes, surfaces, and types of movement with respect to load and overload. The critical limits of a biological material and its behavior under stress are another important aspect of load analysis. This chapter deals with fundamental questions in determining load.

Basically, there are two possibilities to estimate stress in an element of the human body (e.g., in the Achilles tendon or in the ankle joint during jogging): measuring and computing. *Measuring* is the measurement of the relevant variable or an associated quantity from which the relevant variable can be determined. All visible kinematic variables such as angles, accelerations of a marker on the lower limb, pressure distribution underneath the foot during running, and all external force measurements are directly measured variables and belong to this first category.

Computing means to estimate (calculate) the relevant variable using substitutional measurements. In both cases, the terms used describe the variable of interest. For a tendon, for instance, tension describes the force transmitted by the tendon and stress, the force divided by the area of

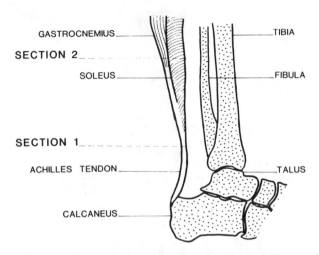

Figure 3.1. Schematic illustration of the tension in the Achilles tendon.

the tendon. In any case, the location of interest must be specified first as illustrated in Figure 3.1 with sections 1 and 2.

A simplification of the reality is shown in Figure 3.2. It is the first step of an abstraction from a real body. Only an ideal or simplified structure can be described by a mechanical, physical, biological, or mathematical model. A model includes some aspects which are of interest from one point of view but excludes other aspects which might be of interest to a researcher studying from another point of view. A model is therefore never complete; however, it is necessary in the case of the computing method approach, which can be characterized as follows:

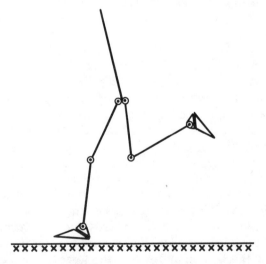

Figure 3.2. Schematic illustration of a model of the human body.

Step 1. Idealization of the human body so that it is possible to determine (estimate) the *relevant variable* with a set of variables which can be measured.

Step 2. Measurement of the variables and calculation of the relevant variable with the model.

A simple but useful idealization of the human body in connection with general questions concerning the lower extremities could be (see Figure 3.2) as follows:

- Forefoot, heel, lower leg, thigh, trunk, including head and upper extremities, are described by rigid bodies with masses m_i and moments of inertia I_i.
- The rigid bodies are connected by joints forming a 9-link model. The joints (in reality, cartilage and ligmaents) are assumed to be ideal and do not change form under stress. Furthermore, the joints are frictionless, and the ligaments are without initial force. The range of motion is not taken into consideration. Such a type of joint is called an *ideal mechanical joint* and is characterized just by the number of degrees of freedom.
- The muscles, including tendons, the force generators of the human body, are assumed as being massless with a cross section which can be neglected. Origins, insertions, and lines of action are known.

Using this idealization, the linked system can be described by the mathematics of *rigid body mechanics*. Note that, in reality, the different segments do not behave like rigid bodies. This is an important aspect during impact. Possibilities taking into account these aspects are reported elsewhere (Nigg & Denoth, 1980; Denoth et al., 1984). Assuming rigid bodies, the problem *load determination/load estimation* is reduced to a mechanical problem.

In rigid body mechanics, there are basically two kinds of approaches: The forces are known and the movement is calculated or vice versa. The first type with known forces involves solving a system of differential equations which is called a *mechanical system*. This type is most frequently seen in mechanics. In load analysis (Paul, 1965; Morrison, 1969; Seireg & Arvikar, 1973; Pedotti et al., 1978; Crowninshield & Brand, 1981) the second approach is more frequent: The movement is known and the internal forces are calculated. However, this second approach is connected with some problems. The muscle forces are not defined only by kinematic variables like muscle length or shortening velocity of the whole muscle. Therefore, the following fundamental lemma is valid in load analysis:

It is impossible to calculate muscle and joint forces based only on the knowledge of the motion if the number of muscles is bigger than the number of degrees of freedom in each joint.

This statement is valid in the dynamic and static case. The solution depends in this context upon the number of degrees of freedom of a joint and the line of action of the different muscle forces. The fact that it is impossible to compute joint forces and muscle forces only with the knowledge of movement represents a fundamental problem. The solution lies in the control system of the force generators.

This fundamental statement is discussed by the example *upper extremities* which are modelled as follows: The upper arm is fixed, the forearm is described by one rigid body, the hand is neglected. Upper arm and forearm are connected by an ideal mechanical joint. The muscles are assumed as being ideal. The biceps brachii (F_{m2}), the brachialis (F_{m3}) and the brachioradialis (F_{m1}) are taken into consideration as flexors. The extensor carpi radialis longus, the pronator, and other muscles are not included in the simple model with one degree of freedom. The equation of motion is:

$$I \ddot{\phi} = \sum_{i=1}^{3} \mathbf{d}_{mi} \times \mathbf{F}_{mi} + \sum_{j=1}^{2} \mathbf{d}_{ej} \times \mathbf{F}_{ej}$$

where: ϕ: coordinate of the forearm with respect to the horizontal line
   I: moment of inertia of the forearm with respect to the hinge joint
   $\mathbf{F}_{mi}$:   muscle force of muscle i (vector)
   $\mathbf{d}_{mi}$:   vector from the joint to the origin of muscle i
   $\mathbf{F}_{ej}$:   external force j (vector)
   $\mathbf{d}_{ej}$:   vector from the joint to the point of application of external force j
   $\times$:   symbol for cross-product (here in two dimensions, therefore: result a scalar).

If the muscle forces are known (as a function of time), and if the external forces describe the acceleration of a rigid body or the deformation of

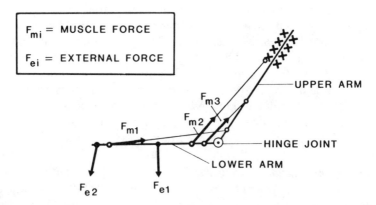

Figure 3.3. Simple model of an arm. The body of interest is the lower arm with two external and three muscle forces acting. All muscle forces in this example are agonists and no antagonist is included in this model.

a spring, then the motion of the forearm can be determined using the equation of motion. However, if the motion of the forearm $\phi(t)$, the external forces, and their points of application are known, as is typically the case in biomechanics, the equation of motion provides only *one* condition for *all* muscles, namely:

$$\sum_{i=1}^{3} \mathbf{d}_{mi} \times \mathbf{F}_{mi} = I\,\ddot{\phi} - \sum_{j=1}^{2} \mathbf{d}_{ej} \times \mathbf{F}_{ej} = M$$

where: M(t) = total moment at the joint produced by all three muscles.

The direction of the muscle forces is a function of the angle ϕ and can be described by the unit vectors $\mathbf{e}_{mi}$. Using this unit vector, the muscle force can be described as:

$$\mathbf{F}_{mi} = F_{mi}\,\mathbf{e}_{mi}(\phi)$$

This shows that a linear relationship exists between the magnitude of the muscle force and the moment M at each time:

$$\sum_{i=1}^{3} d_{mi}\,F_{mi} = M$$

where: $d_{mi} = \mathbf{d}_{mi} \times \mathbf{e}_{mi}$

Therefore, it is not possible to determine the three muscle forces only from the equation of motion. Because the force in the joint depends upon the individual muscle forces, it is impossible to compute the stress in the joint. The linear relationship between the three muscles represents a plane in a three-dimensional space (Figure 3.4). Because the individual muscle forces are not negative, the solution must lie in the range (0, M/d_{mi}). If no upper limits of muscle forces are taken into account, then each point

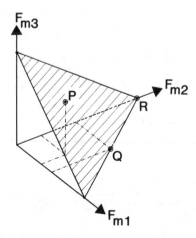

Figure 3.4. The linear relationship between the three muscle forces at one time t_i. P, Q, and R illustrate three possible solutions discussed later.

inside the triangle (M/d_{m1}, M/d_{m2}, M/d_{m3}) is a possible solution for the muscle forces. Point P, for instance, represents a solution where all three muscles are active; point Q, a solution without activity of the third muscle; and point R, a solution where only the second muscle is working. Without more information, the "correct" solution—out of an infinite number—cannot be determined. The additional information can be supplied from various fields. Aspects of the control system in a muscle model could come from fields such as physiology and neurology. EMG signals are often used in this context to give an idea of possible solutions. However, at present, most models use the approach of a unique solution without considering the control system of the force generators. In the following some possible strategies are discussed briefly:

SIMPLIFY THE MODEL (REDUCTION)

The model is constructed in a way that the number of muscles included provide a unique solution of the problem (Paul, 1965; Morrison, 1969; Procter, 1980; Baumann & Stucke, 1980). The above example of the arm could just include one muscle. The muscle force computed from the given motion then is:

$$F_m(t) = M(t)/d_m(t)$$

However, the example of the arm as illustrated in Figure 3.3 is, with respect to the number of muscles, already a simplification of reality because not all agonists and no antagonists are included. Therefore, this approach provides an idea of the order of magnitude of the force of such a muscle group represented by F_m.

THE SOLUTION HAS TO FULFILL ADDITIONAL CONSTRAINTS

The muscle and/or the joint forces have to fulfill additional conditions (Seireg & Arvikar, 1973; Pedotti et al., 1978; Crowninshield & Brand, 1981). They may be based on mathematical techniques and/or physiological principles. Some appear to be more and others less physiological. Examples of such approaches are as follows:

1. The forces per cross-sectional area in all muscles involved are equal.

$$F_{mi}/A_i = \lambda(t), i = 1,2,\ldots$$

where: A_i = cross-sectional area of muscle m_i

2. The sum of all muscle forces is a minimum.

$$\sum_{i=1}^{n} F_{mi} = minimum$$

3. The sum of all muscle tensions is a minimum or, more general, the sum of all muscle tensions to the power p is a minimum.

$$\sum_{i=1}^{n} (F_{mi}/A_i)^p = \text{minimum}$$

The first approach gives a result where all muscles are working. This corresponds to point P in Figure 3.4. Linear conditions (Approach 2 and 3 with p = 1) have solutions (if a unique solution exists) where only one muscle is active. This corresponds to corner points in Figure 3.4. Approach 3, with p > 1, provides results where all muscles are active. The first special constraint, $F_{mi}/A_i = \lambda(t)$, includes (at least in a static or quasistatic case) some physiological aspects. However, different fiber types (slow and fast) are not taken into account. Therefore, the stress in all muscles is the same. If the nervous control system really did work in such a way, dynamically, and for all muscle fibers, no muscle strain could occur. However, in reality, muscle strain is found in sport activities. Constraints, including economy aspects (Denoth, 1982), increase the complexity of the problem.

NO UNIQUE SOLUTION

If the model is not too complex, the solution space can be discussed. For the example with the arm (Figure 3.3), the solutions are characterized by two parameters, α and β, and the muscle force of muscle m_i is described at any time by:

$$F_{mi}(\alpha,\beta) = \lambda_i^2 M/d_{mi}$$
$$i = 1, 2, 3$$

with $\quad \lambda_1 = \sin \alpha \cos \beta$
$\qquad \lambda_2 = \sin \alpha \sin \beta$
$\qquad \lambda_3 = \cos \alpha$

The joint force as a function of α and β is described by:

$$F_j (\alpha,\beta) = m\ddot{x} - F_e - M \sum_{i=1}^{3} \lambda_i^2 e_{mi}/d_{mi}$$

A comparison between the *no unique solution* and the *additional constraints* approach shows the advantages and disadvantages of the different strategies. An approach with additional constraints has the advantage to give one solution for a force in an element of interest. However, the result very much depends on the constraints used. In contrast, the no unique solution approach does not provide a number but a set of possible solutions, which can be used to discuss various possibilities. One can, for instance, check what forces would act if only one muscle would work, possibly getting a more comprehensive understanding of the problems. This may be of importance in the analysis of pain and injuries.

WITH CONTROL SYSTEM

The nervous control system works in a complex pattern even for simple every day movements such as gait or running. Many aspects of this ingenious computer system are still unknown. Myocybernetic control models were used by Hatze (1981) in order to describe human movement. Other aspects of a control system are described by Pierrynowski (1982) and Denoth (1983). However, in load analysis this step of introducing a control system has not yet been included. Our own approach of including the aspect of a control system is explained in the following:

Each control system or regulator is characterized (besides many other factors) by the latent period T_l. External impact forces have a relatively short time duration. If the duration of the impact T_i is smaller than the latent period T_l, then the control system is unable to react and to change the level of activity during this impact (Nigg & Denoth, 1980). During this impact phase, the muscles can be described as independent force generators. The muscle force depends upon the active state (Hatze, 1981) or the intrinsic state (Hill, 1970) and the length and the velocity of the contractile element. Therefore, the problem, calculation of muscle forces, can theoretically be solved during the "impact phase." The EMG signal provides a rough estimation of the intrinsic state of a muscle (not the force) in such a situation.

The outlined problems in connection with theoretical load analysis can easily be expanded. They illustrate the complexity of such an approach. However, they should not discourage an attempt to improve theoretical considerations. On the contrary, theoretical considerations should be studied with more intensity to provide more understanding and quantitative information with respect to load and stress on the human body during movements such as running and jogging.

Measurements of external forces can be performed with little problem (see chapter 2). Furthermore, it is possible to calculate the joint moments produced by all the muscles acting (Pedotti et al., 1978; Winter, 1983, 1984; Capozzo, 1984). The comments in this chapter suggest that there are many more problems if one tries to quantify internal forces. In this case, two main hurdles are to be overcome. On one side, the anthropometrical information has to be included. Lines of action, origins, lengths, and other individual information have to be determined and used in the calculations. This can be done (e.g., Pierynowski, 1982) and the calculated forces will be more or less accurate depending on the method used. Therefore, this problem is solved. There is also the basic problem that, from a mathematical point of view, the musculoskeletal system is undetermined. There are more muscles than needed to execute a certain movement which results, in a mathematical sense, in too many unknowns or not enough equations. The final decision, which of the possible strategies to choose, depends on the question under investigation. If the order of magnitude of the forces in the hip joint is of interest, a reduction approach, as used by Paul (1965), is appropriate. However, in the analysis of pain and injuries, the reduction method may probably not be applied because the single elements are important. In this case, a no unique solution approach, or an approach with a control system may provide the best results.

The Transfer Function: External to Internal Variables

Ground reaction force or kinematic variables such as angular position, velocity, angular velocity, and accleration are usually used in gait analysis to describe the movements. Reasons why force curves or movement patterns have a certain shape are discussed in connection with pain, injury pattern, or anatomical abnormalities. The conclusions are due merely to results of statistical analyses or may sometimes represent projections made by the scientist. Fundamental statements concerning the load on the locomotor system due to external variables are discussed in this chapter, which also gives some information about the order of magnitude of internal forces and the factors influencing load in the locomotor system. A reduction approach is therefore used in the following examples. The main interest is to know the shape of this transfer function (external to internal variables) in walking or running, or, as an example, which variables are needed to calculate, for instance, the force exerted at the ankle joint. Note that the main emphasis lies in the use of the basic principles and in the simplicity of the used models.

In the first example, the forces at the ankle joint and at the Achilles tendon during the stance-phase of walking are discussed. In the second example, the subtalar joint will be included. A mechanical model describing the impact at touch down during jogging is discussed in the third example. The fourth example discusses external and internal forces in a model which includes a foot using the results of the third example. In these four examples, only forces are calculated. Naturally, these forces are transferred to the segments of the body, which implies a knowledge of the geometry of the body to calculate the real stress. In Examples 5 and 6, the calculation of stress distribution in the Achilles tendon and in a hinge joint is illustrated.

FORCES IN THE ANKLE JOINT (EXAMPLE 1)

We simplify the lower extremities and make the following assumptions: Both foot and shank are rigid bodies connected by an ideal mechanical hinge joint (Figure 3.5). The movement is restrained to the saggital plane which is assumed to be perpendicular to the joint axis. The muscles which move the foot with respect to the shank are represented by two idealized

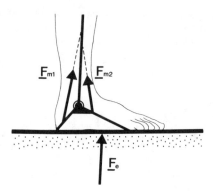

Figure 3.5. Simple model of foot and lower leg.

muscles, an agonist and an antagonist (F_{m1}, F_{m2}). The two muscles are mutually controlled so that they never produce force simultaneously. If co-contraction is included, the stress on muscles, bones, cartilage, and so forth is increased. In this example, a quasistatic estimation of the forces is performed. The transfer problem, therefore, reduces to an estimation of the time history of the lever arms with respect to the axis of the upper ankle joint. The lever arms are the distance of the force application lines of the two muscles (d_1 and d_2) and of the external force (d), all with respect to the joint. The sign of the generated moment is assigned to the distances. In this example, d_1 is always positive and d_2 negative. The distance d changes the sign. It is positive at heel contact and negative at toe-off. Quasistatic considerations lead to the equations:

if $d > 0$ $\mathbf{F}_{m2} + \mathbf{F}_e + \mathbf{F}_j = 0$
        $F_{m2}d_2 + F_e d = 0,$
if $d < 0$ $\mathbf{F}_{m1} + \mathbf{F}_e + \mathbf{F}_j = 0$
        $F_{m1}d_1 + F_e d = 0$
where $\mathbf{F}_j$ = joint force.

The force produced by Muscle 1 (the force transmitted by the Achilles tendon) according to these equations is:

$F_{m1} = 0$ if $d > 0$ heel contact

$F_{m1} = \dfrac{(-d)}{d_1} F_e$ if $d < 0$ toe-off

The force at the joint is:

$\mathbf{F}_j = -\mathbf{F}_e - \mathbf{F}_{m2}$ if $d > 0$
$\mathbf{F}_j = -\mathbf{F}_e - \mathbf{F}_{m1}$ if $d < 0$

The force at the Achilles tendon is always zero in this simplified model if the external force $\mathbf{F}_e$ exerts a positive moment. The relative position of foot and shank determine both the directions of the muscle forces F_{m1} and F_{m2} and the distances d_1 and d_2. The distance d depends upon the coordinate of the center of pressure, the coordinate of the pivot, and the direction of the external force. These distances can be determined if force and film measurements are made simultaneously. In order to estimate an order of magnitude of the forces in the joint and the muscle forces, we discuss the *stance-phase*. In this case, the sole of the foot is assumed to be parallel to the floor, and the change in position of the lower leg is small. Therefore, the distances d_1 and d_2 are nearly constant. The horizontal forces are neglected for this example. This is not without some problems which will be discussed in the final comments for this example. The distance d is defined by the center of pressure point k. The distance heel-ball in a normal step is $k_{max} - k_{min} = \Delta k$. In addition, we assume that the distance ratio for heel-projection pivot to projection pivot-ball is 1:3 as illustrated in Figure 3.6.

These assumptions (simplifications) provide enough knowledge to determine from the measured reaction, force in the vertical direction F_z and its center of pressure, the transfer to the internal variables. The corresponding formulas are:

$$k < 0 \qquad F_{m1} = 0 \qquad\qquad F_{m2} = F_z \frac{k}{d_2}$$

$$k > 0 \qquad F_{m1} = F_z \frac{k}{d_1} \qquad F_{m2} = 0$$

For the magnitude of the resultant joint forces:

$$k < 0 \qquad F_j \sim F_z(1 - \frac{k}{d_2})$$

$$k > 0 \qquad F_j \sim F_z(1 - \frac{k}{d_1})$$

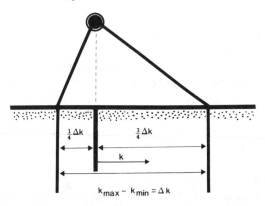

Figure 3.6. Assumptions used for the estimation of forces in the Achilles tendon and ankle joint. k is the coordinate of the center of pressure, k is zero underneath the joint, positive in the forefoot, and negative in the rearfoot.

Figure 3.7 schematically shows the calculated forces at joint and tendon for the same reaction force but different application history. The example illustrates that it is not possible to predict muscle and joint forces by using only ground reaction forces. It is a clear illustration of the importance of the geometry in the estimation of internal forces. The time dependency of the center of pressure has a significant influence on the load of the muscles and the ankle joint. Similar estimations can be made for heel-strike and toe-off.

COMMENTS ON EXAMPLE 1

1. The geometrical configuration is important for the prediction of muscle forces (see chapter 1). Changes in the movement pattern are always connected with changes in the internal forces. Therefore, if the internal forces are the variables of interest, models have to be used to estimate these forces.
2. The example in Figure 3.7 is a schematic illustration. The curves for the center of pressure path are exaggerated. In reality, curves like the dash-dot line are most unlikely. In most of the cases analyzed, the path of the center of pressure curve is above the straight line, and the variation in the joint and tendon forces are smaller. However, this does not reduce the importance of the influence of geometry. Once again, these examples have the purpose to improve the basic understanding and not to provide accurate numbers. In this case, the new knowledge is the importance of the geometry. This example (as well as the following examples) illustrates that measurement of external forces is one thing and estimation of internal forces is another thing. It is impossible to deduce from exclusive external ground reaction force measurements the internal forces without additional information on the geometry. It illustrates the danger of material test and the transfer of such results into load analysis during running if such tests do not include the geometry.
3. The calculations in this example were made neglecting the influence of the horizontal components. However, the total moment produced by the ground reaction force with respect to the joint is sensitive to the height of the joint and, therefore, to the height of the heel. In order to take this aspect into account, the a-p force must be included. This moment due to the a-p force component can, at some points in time, easily be bigger than the moment produced by the vertical component because both change signs during stance-phase but at different times.
4. The forces in the Achilles tendon during walking can easily reach 2 to 3 times body weight. The forces in the joint are slightly higher as illustrated in Figure 3.7 and discussed in Table 1.3.

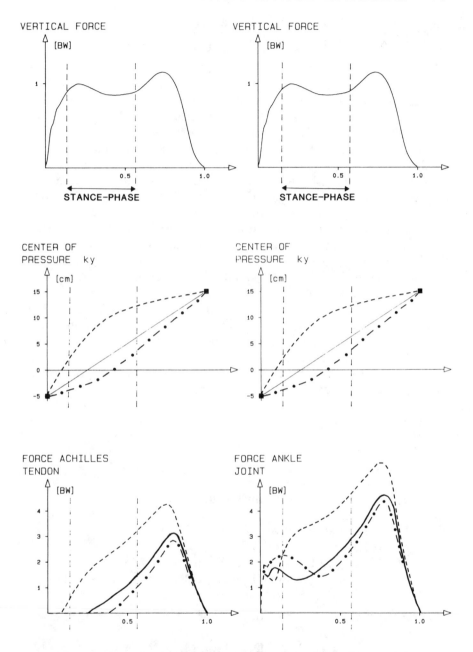

Figure 3.7. Comparison of external vertical ground reaction force and force in the Achilles tendon and in the joint, using a simple model for a quasi-static situation with d_1 = 5 cm for walking. The results between the two slashed lines illustrate stance-phase for which the model was developed.

FORCES IN THE ACHILLES TENDON, ANKLE, AND SUBTALAR JOINT (EXAMPLE 2)

Foot and shank are simplified as two rigid bodies in analogy to the first example. They are connected by two ideal mechanical hinge joints. The talus located between these two joints is assumed as being massless. The axes of the two joints (Axis 1—ankle joint; Axis 2—subtalar joint) are not parallel. Therefore, the motion of the foot with respect to the shank is not restricted to one plane. The muscular system is represented by four idealized muscles (m_1, m_2, m_3, m_4). Muscle m_1 and muscle m_2 are the main muscles responsible for the movement around the ankle joint and are defined in the same way as for Example 1. Muscle m_3 and muscle m_4 have the same function for the subtalar joint. The lines of action of the four muscles and the axes of the two joints are aligned in a way that each muscle generates a moment with respect to both axes. It is assumed that the neural control system acts analogous to Example 1: Agonist and antagonist never exert their force simultaneously. Using this assumption, the stress estimated with this model for muscles, tendons, cartilage, and bones is a minimum estimation. If co-contraction were considered, the real values would be higher. However, results from the literature (Pierrynowski, 1982) suggest that the influence of co-contraction is relatively small for the foot region.

In the quasistatic case, the motion of the rigid body "foot" is described by the following equations of equilibrium:

$$\sum_{i=1}^{4} \mathbf{F}_{mi} + \mathbf{F}_e + \mathbf{F}_{j2} = 0$$

$$\sum_{i=1}^{4} \mathbf{d}_{mi} \times \mathbf{F}_{mi} + \mathbf{d}_e \times \mathbf{F}_e + \mathbf{M}_e + \mathbf{d}_{j2} \times \mathbf{F}_{j2} + \mathbf{M}_{j2} = 0$$

with $\mathbf{F}_{mi}$ = muscle forces of muscle mi
$\mathbf{F}_e$ = external force
$\mathbf{F}_{j2}$ = resultant force at the subtalar joint
$\mathbf{M}_e$ = external moment
$\mathbf{M}_{j2}$ = moment transmitted through the subtalar joint
$\mathbf{d}$ = distances (vectors) from the center of mass of the foot to the points of application of the forces.

The transfer problem is again reduced to an estimation of the lever arms.

$$\sum_{i=1}^{4} \mathbf{D}_{mi} \times \mathbf{F}_{mi} + \mathbf{D}_e \times \mathbf{F}_e + \mathbf{M}_e + \mathbf{M}_{j2} = 0$$

where $\mathbf{D}_{mi} = \mathbf{d}_{mi} - \mathbf{d}_{j2}$
$\mathbf{D}_e = \mathbf{d}_e - \mathbf{d}_{j2}$

The component of the moment M_{j2} at the subtalar joint in direction of the axis itself is zero because the joint is assumed to be an ideal mechanical joint. Therefore, the equation for this component is:

$$\sum_{i=1}^{4} (\mathbf{D}_{mi} \times \mathbf{F}_{mi}) \cdot \mathbf{e}_{j2} + (\mathbf{D}_e \times \mathbf{F}_e) \cdot \mathbf{e}_{j2} + \mathbf{M}_e \cdot \mathbf{e}_{j2} = 0$$

This means that for the projected vectors into the plane perpendicular to the axis of the subtalar joint similar equations hold as in the first example, namely:

$$\sum_{i=1}^{4} d_i F_{mi} + d_e F_e + M_e = 0$$

where: F_{mi}: muscle force of muscle mi
   d_i: distance of the projected muscle force from the Axis 2 (subtalar joint)
   F_e: external force
   d_e: distance (perpendicular) of projected external forces from Axis 2
   M_e: projected external moment with respect to Axis 2

with $\mathbf{F}_{mi} = F_{mi}\mathbf{e}_{mi}$
   $d_i = (\mathbf{D}_{mi} \times \mathbf{e}_{mi}) \cdot \mathbf{e}_{j2}$

Similar equations result for the ankle joint. Using the assumption that only one muscle per joint is active (no antagonistic activity), one can estimate muscle and joint forces as described by Procter (1980). This approach is basically not different compared to the approach used in Example 1. The main difference is the use of 3-D input. The difference which is interesting for running shoe analysis is the use of both coordinates of the center of pressure k_x and k_y, because the path of the center of pressure (Figure 3.8) can easily be influenced by shoe construction.

COMMENTS ON EXAMPLE 2

1. The time history and the geometrical path of the center of pressure and, therefore, the stress can be influenced by sport shoes (Nigg & Luethi, 1980). If, for example, the stress in Muscle 3 is too high (a result based on a medical diagnosis), the stress in this muscle can be reduced by changing the path of the center of pressure. The path of the center of pressure should change so that the lever arm between external force and subtalar joint changes to a less curved line which would result in a reduction of the force (stress) in Muscle 3. Note that the concept is not to reduce the external forces. Rather than changing the magnitude of the force, one tries to change the point of application in order

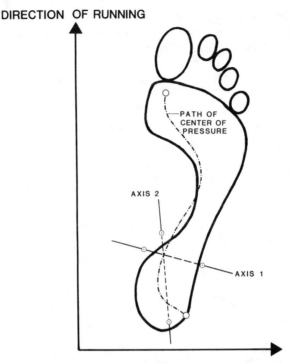

Figure 3.8. Schematic illustration of the center of pressure relative to the two axes.

to reduce the moment. This is a very important concept for shoe construction.

2. This example illustrates, again, that the combination between external measurements, force, center of pressure, film, and modelling provides specific information with respect to strategies to use when pain occurs. This approach is more analytical and based less on speculation. It allows us to study a specific problem and to suggest solutions for this problem.

3. There is no doubt that the ideal solution for load analysis consists in the use of film and force measurements together with a model. However, it is possible to use only force platform information (force and center of pressure) if simplified assumptions are used. The procedure would be similar to Example 1. The foot would geometrically be subdivided in four regions (Figure 3.8). Such an approach is, of course, not as comprehensive as a film/force approach but provides more information than isolated force analysis.

IMPACT FOOT-SURFACE (EXAMPLE 3)

The explanations in Examples 1 and 2 are based on a quasistatic approximation. Such an approximation obviously cannot be used for impact

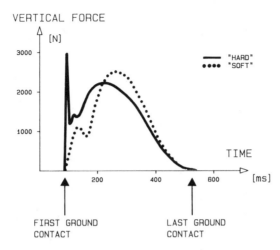

Figure 3.9. Example of the vertical component of the ground reaction force for running on two very different surfaces.

problems. However, an impact occurs each time the foot (chapter 1) contacts the surface during walking or running. The impact heel-surface, heel-shoe-surface, or toe-surface during walking, jogging, or jumping can easily be illustrated with the ground reaction force (Figures 1.9 and 1.10). Shoe material and shoe geometry may influence these peaks. In a general and very simplified way, one could say, The softer the material, the larger the deceleration distance and, therefore, the smaller the impact force (if the initial and boundary conditions remain constant).

The vertical component of the ground reaction force for a very soft and a very hard surface during jogging (a real heel-jogger) is illustrated in Figure 3.10. The impact force amplitude on the hard surface is about 2.5 times the corresponding amplitude for the soft one. During the stance phase, however, the ground reaction force is slightly higher for the softer material. This result is expected if the movement of the center of mass for both surfaces is equal during the flight phase. If the position of the foot for these two shoe types is the same, then the stress of muscles and joints is about 20% higher for the softer surface in the stance-phase (active part of the force-curve). Note that this example is for extreme materials. In reality the differences in the active peak are very small for the hardnesses used for running shoes as illustrated in Table 2.7. These numbers show an average difference between shore 25 and 45 of only 18 N for different velocities which is less than 1%. There is a big difference in the impact peak between the two surfaces, and it is of general interest to understand the relationship between impact peak and load or stress in joints, muscles, or tendons. Furthermore, it is important to know the factors which influence the impact peak and how this impact can be described mechanically.

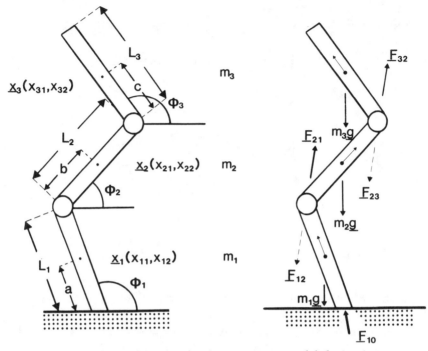

Figure 3.10. Free body diagram of a three-segment model during impact.

The reaction force due to an impact of a rigid body (iron shot, e.g., with different materials) shows a similar shape of force peak or impact peak as in walking or jogging (see Figure 1.8), which is not surprising. The impact between a rigid body and a deformable material is easy to describe mechanically. In the simplest model,

- the material behaves like an ideal spring (linear);
- the contact area between body and material is a constant; and
- the gravitational force is neglected.

This results in a harmonic oscillator:

$$m\ddot{x} + fx = 0$$

where: m: mass
x: coordinate of the center of mass
f: spring constant

The solution of this simple differential equation with the initial conditions:

$x(0) = 0$ and
$\dot{x}(0) = -v$ and $v > 0$

is

$$x(t) = -\frac{v}{\Omega} \sin \Omega\, t$$

with $\Omega^2 = \dfrac{f}{m}$

The maximum reaction force or the impact peak is:

$$F_{max} = F_{zi} = vm\Omega = v\sqrt{fm}$$

and depends upon the impact velocity, the mass of the rigid body, and the hardness of the material.

Therefore, the softer the material of surface or shoe, the smaller is the impact peak if the material is thick enough. The result indicates that the impact velocity has the greatest influence on the amplitude of the impact peak (expressed in percent). This impact velocity depends on the runner's style and can be influenced. However, the locomotor system itself is a system of many rigid and nonrigid bodies. Therefore, the simplification of the human body to a single rigid body may create problems and may not be adequate. It is, for instance, not evident how big the mass m of this single rigid body should be. Is it the mass of a foot or the mass of the whole body?

In order to increase the understanding of the impact "human body-surface" in selected sport activities with a marked heel contact, the behavior of a three-segment model (Figure 3.10) during impact is discussed. The first segment represents the shank and the foot (without an ankle joint), the second segment the thigh, and the third segment the rest of the body. All three segments are assumed to be rigid, however, with a reduced mass. This reduced mass includes contributions from the nonrigid mass of muscles, fat, and so forth (Denoth et al., 1985). The three segments are connected by two ideal mechanical hinge joints. The motion is restricted to a plane. Muscles as force generators are not introduced because we are only investigating the impact. The estimated joint forces, therefore, will generally be smaller than in reality (Denoth, 1983). The dynamic behavior of such a kinematic chain is defined by the set of differential equations:

$$m_1\ddot{x}_1 = m_1g + F_{10} + F_{12}$$
$$m_2\ddot{x}_2 = m_2g + F_{21} + F_{23}$$
$$m_3\ddot{x}_3 = m_3g + F_{32}$$
$$I_1\ddot{\phi}_1 = -ae(\phi_1) \times F_{10} + (L_1 - a)e(\phi_1) \times F_{12}$$
$$I_2\ddot{\phi}_2 = -be(\phi_2) \times F_{21} + (L_2 - b)e(\phi_2) \times F_{23}$$
$$I_3\ddot{\phi}_3 = -ce(\phi_3) \times F_{32}$$

The constraints are:

$$x_2 = x_1 + (L_1 - a)e(\phi_1) + be(\phi_2)$$
$$x_3 = x_2 + (L_2 - b)e(\phi_2) + ce(\phi_3)$$

with ϕ_i = angle of the element i in relation to the horizontal line measured at the posterior side

L_i = length of the rigid body i
    a, b, c are the distances between the distal end of the element and the center of mass

x_i = vector from the origin of the center of mass of element i
    $x_1 = (x_{11}, x_{12})$
    $x_2 = (x_{21}, x_{22})$
    $x_3 = (x_{31}, x_{32})$
    where the first index indicates the element and the second the direction

m_i = mass of the element

I_i = moment of inertia of the element i with respect to the center of mass

$m_i g$ = gravitation force of the element i

F_{10} = ground reaction force

F_{ik} = joint reaction force, force at the element i due to the element k

The ground reaction force F_{10} is defined by the components in the x and z direction. The component in the z-direction describes the material properties of the surface/shoe/heel system, and is a function of the deformation and velocity of the material. The component in the x-direction describes the friction characteristics of the heel/shoe/surface system. This system of differential equations is not linear. Solutions are found by iteration with the help of the computer.

Calculations with the model show (unpublished results, Denoth) that, under certain conditions, the 3-link model with five degrees of freedom can be reduced to a system of one degree of freedom with a defined *effective mass* m^*. The effective mass is a weighted mean value of the quotient

$$Q(t) = \frac{F_{10}}{|\ddot{x}_1 + g|}$$

Such an effective mass can only be used if this mass remains relatively constant or if possible changes are known. In order to illustrate the time dependency, we define time points in the force-time diagram. t_{max} is defined as the time when $F = F_{max}$, $t_{+1/2}$ as the time when F decreased to $1/2 F_{max}$ after t_{max} and $t_{-1/2}$ as the time when F reaches $1/2 F_{max}$ on the increasing side. The result from the 3-link model shows that the effective mass is relatively constant for knee angles between 90 and 140° (see Figure 3.11).

The values for the mass for the time period before the maximum is reached is too small and afterward too high. For higher knee angles, the differences are between 5% and about 15%. However, one can state that the effective mass is relatively constant during the time around the impact peak. Therefore, the description of the effective mass is acceptable because $Q(t)$ does not vary much during the impact.

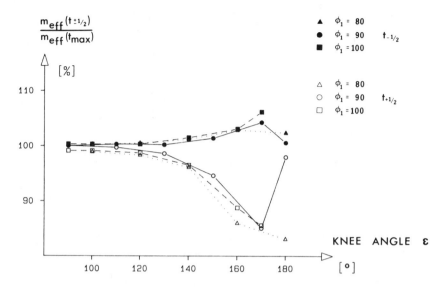

Figure 3.11. Changes in the effective mass during impact for different initial conditions.

In conclusion, the ground reaction force at touch down of a 3-link model can be approximated by the impact of a rigid body with a known effective mass. For this effective mass m^* (or m_{eff}), the equation of motion by Newton in (more or less) the vertical direction is given by:

$$m^* \ddot{z} = F - m^* g$$

The effective mass m^* is basically a function of the three segmental masses m_1, m_2, and m_3, the initial conditions, and the characteristics of the surface. One important variable in sport activities such as walking, running, and jumping is the angle of the knee. This influence is illustrated in Figure 3.12.

The effective mass can be used to estimate reaction forces in walking and running. The reaction force depends on the factors:

- effective mass: m^*
- impact velocity: $-v$
- stiffness of the ground: f

The true equation of motion of the shank in the vertical direction is:

$$m_1 \ddot{z} = F_{10} + F_{12} - m_1 g$$

The approximated equation using the effective mass is:

$$m^* \ddot{z} = F_{10} - m^* g$$

Consequently, the impact force at the knee joint is given by:

$$F_{12} = -(m^* - m_1)(\ddot{z} + g)$$

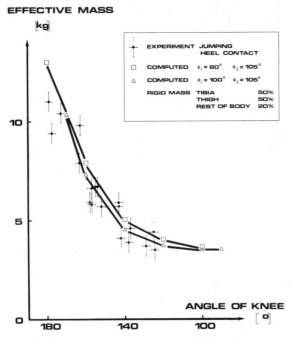

Figure 3.12. Results of the effective mass as a function of the knee angle from the 3-link model and from experiments for a test subject with the mass of 65 kg (barefoot).

or

$$F_{12} = -\frac{m^* - m_1}{m^*} F_{10}$$

These calculations illustrate that the effective mass can be useful to describe the impact force at the knee. Example: The variable of interest is the impact force at the knee joint; the knee angle and the acceleration of the shank or the ground reaction force can be measured. Using these measured external variables, the impact force amplitudes can be estimated as illustrated in Table 3.1.

COMMENTS ON EXAMPLE 3

1. The results in Table 3.1 indicate that both ground reaction force and acceleration, as isolated results, occurring during human movement do not provide an insight into joint forces. Both ground reaction forces showed the same amplitude in the examples used. However, the forces in the knee joint are different. This is, once more, an indication of how important the combination of the external measurements with a model is.

Table 3.1. Estimation of impact force peaks with the help of the effective mass.

Movement	Measured				Calculated	
	v_0 (m/s)	ϵ_0 (°)	a (m/s²)	F_{10} (N)	m* (kg)	F_{21} (N)
Running heel-toe (barefoot)						
Case 1	−1.0	165	200	—	8	1100
Case 2	−1.0	165	—	1600	8	1100
Landing on surface in gymnasium (crouch position)						
Case 1	−1.4	130	400	—	4	1600
Case 2	−1.4	130	—	1600	4	1600

2. Mechanically, the quality of the model of the effective mass can be improved by introducing a tensor. However, the basic finding will not change (unpublished results, Denoth & Ruder).
3. The model does not include muscles. Some justification for this approach is discussed in chapter 1 (Figure 1.11). The activity of muscles is considered as having a limited influence on the impact force peaks. However, the effect of muscles is that they basically increase the joint forces (Denoth, 1985).
4. The three-segment model was developed to increase the understanding of impact forces. In this first attempt, the foot was neglected. However, it must be included for a more detailed analysis.
5. The results for impact forces and knee angle are very much subject and shoe/surface dependent. The values in Figure 3.12 are for barefoot and a subject with m = 65 kg. The values for running with running shoes are higher because the loading rate is smaller.
6. The effective mass depends heavily on the time characteristics of the impact force. It is increasing with decreasing frequency of the impact force.

IMPACT FORCES AND GEOMETRY OF THE FOOT (EXAMPLE 4)

The path of the center of pressure is influenced by the shoe as explained earlier. The transfer from external to internal forces is influenced by this path, and it is, therefore, logical to use a model which includes the foot in order to quantify internal impact forces. A simple model which enables one to estimate internal impact forces is illustrated in Figure 3.13. It consists of a rigid foot, an effective mass, and a muscle in the medial part of the foot. Because the impact forces in running are dominant in the vertical direction, only this component is discussed. The two horizontal com-

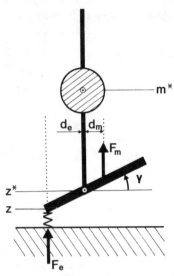

Figure 3.13. Simple model for the estimation of internal impact forces in walking and running (rear view of a left foot).

ponents are neglected and the lower leg is assumed to remain in the vertical position. The symbols used are as follows:

m_f = mass of foot
m^* = effective mass of rest of the body
I = moment of inertia of foot
F_e = vertical component of ground reaction force
F_j = vertical component of joint force
F_m = muscle force
z = coordinate of the heel
z_f = coordinate of foot
z^* = coordinate of m^*
d_f = distance between center of mass of the foot and joint
d_e = distance between F_e and joint
d_m = distance between F_m and joint
γ = rearfoot angle

The formal solution is:

$$m_f \ddot{z}_f = F_e - F_j + F_m$$
$$m^* \ddot{z}^* = F_j - F_m$$
$$I\ddot{\gamma} - d_f m_f \ddot{z}_f = -d_e F_e + d_m F_m$$

For small angles γ we can write

$$d_e, d_m \cong \text{constant and}$$
$$z_f = z + (d_e - d_f)\, \gamma$$
$$z^* = z + d_e \gamma$$

For the surface/shoe we assume for simplicity

$$F_e = -fz$$

This leads (for $d_f = 0$) to the equation of motion for the heel-coordinate z

$$(m^* + m_f)\ddot{z} = -fz(1 + \frac{(m^* + m_f) \, d_e^2}{I}) - \frac{(m^* + m_f)d_e d_m}{I} F_m$$

In the following, we discuss two special cases: the first where no motion in the subtalar joint is allowed, and the second where movement is allowed. The first special case where $\ddot{\gamma} = 0$ and $\dot{\gamma}_0 = 0$ provides the following results for external and internal impact peak:

external:

$$F_{emax} = F_{zi} = f\frac{z_0}{\Omega_0} = f\frac{v_0}{\Omega_0}$$

with $\Omega_0^2 = \dfrac{f}{m^* + m} \approx \dfrac{f}{m^*}$

internal:

$$F_{jmax} \cong (1 + \frac{d_e}{d_m}) \, F_{emax}$$

The calculations for the second case where movement in the subtalar joint is possible provides the following general results for external impact peaks and internal forces:

external:

$$F_e = f\frac{v_0}{\Omega} \sin\Omega t + \Omega_0^2 \frac{(m^* + m_f)d_e d_m}{I} \int_0^t \frac{\sin\Omega(t - t')}{\Omega} F_m(t')dt'$$

with $\Omega = c \cdot \Omega_0$

and $c^2 = 1 + (m^* + m_f)d_e^2/I$

internal:

$$F_j \cong (1 - \frac{m_f d_f d_e}{I + m_f d_f^2})F_e + (1 + \frac{m_f d_f d_m}{I + m_f d_f^2})F_m$$

COMMENTS ON EXAMPLE 4

1. A comparison of the externally measured impact forces $F_{emax} = F_{zi}$ shows two interesting results: The external impact peak F_{zi} in the case where movement (pronation) is occurring can never exceed the corresponding values for no movement; furthermore, the result shows that impact force peaks measured with a force platform must be smaller for shoes where the first contact is on the outside than for shoes where the landing occurs more under the heel if the muscle force remains constant. Note that muscle force and muscle activity are not the same. It is, therefore, expected that shoes with a positive flare have lower impact forces than shoes with a rounded lateral heel part (negative flare)

if all other conditions are kept constant. An estimation of the influence of the lever arm shows that the external force peak (first peak) decreases with increasing lever arm d_e with a factor of about $\sqrt{1 + 3d_e^2}$. These theoretical considerations are supported by experimental evidence. Denoth et al. (1984) and Kaelin et al. (1984) showed that the external impact force peaks did not change for shoes with shore values between 30 and 60. This result is in agreement with results illustrated in Table 2.7 and Figure 5.6. The result could be explained with a change in the lever arm (smaller for soft and bigger for hard).

An additional support for the results of this model are unpublished experimental data (from Nigg) with a shoe with a rounded heel and another shoe with a heel with a flare of about 15°. The external impact peak showed clearly higher values for the rounded heel. However, the difference was smaller than one would expect due to the change of the lever arm d_e. The control of the initial conditions showed that the landing velocity of the heel of the rounded shoe was about 25% smaller compared to the shoe with the flare. An adaptation effect did obviously occur.

2. The ground reaction forces and the joint forces obtained from model simulations for different levers are shown in Figure 3.14. The muscle is described by a contractile and a series elastic element. Antagonistic muscle activity (co-contraction) is included in these simulations. The pretension of the muscles is set to 500 N each.

The graphical illustration shows many results which are important for the basic understanding of shoe construction and impact forces (e.g., ground reaction forces and joint forces are decreasing with increasing levers). The change in levers is also influencing the basic shape of the force-time curves. Furthermore, it can be seen that generally impact forces in the joint increase with increasing external forces. However, the degree of increase depends on the lever arm. The logical consequence of this is that wide heels can be used to control internal joint forces and keep them on a low level. Muscle forces, however, are increasing in this case. It is evident that the knowledge of the external ground reaction force and the lever arm enable one to determine the impact peak in the joint. The procedure is basically clear. The problems lie in the accuracy of the lever arm. It depends on the location of the center of pressure and the joint. Force platforms provide the center of pressure information. However, the center of pressure is just at the beginning of contact very inaccurate. Anyone who has worked with such systems will appreciate this problem. The determination of the location of the joint may even produce more problems because it is not an ideal joint. In conclusion, it seems to be easier to provide the theoretical background as illustrated in Figure 3.14 than to apply this knowledge in a real experimental set-up.

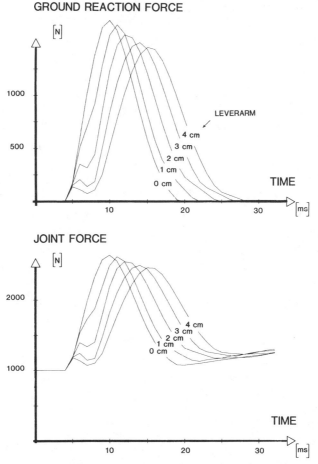

Figure 3.14. Ground reaction forces (top) and joint forces (bottom) obtained from model simulations for different levers (d_e = 0, 1, 2, 3, 4 cm, γ° = 5°).

3. The internal impact forces in joints should not be studied in an isolated manner. Moments produced by external forces and lever arms have certainly an influence on the loading of supporting structures such as ligaments and muscles on the medial side. An increase in the lever arm most likely produces an increase in the angular velocity of the rear-foot ($\dot{\gamma}$) which is proportional to the loading rate of the ligaments, tendons, and muscles. Generally formulated, a decrease in the internal impact peaks in the joint is connected with an increase in the loading rate of the supporting structures if nothing else is changed. For this reason, other strategies should be studied to control and decrease pronation while maintaining the advantage of a reasonable flare with respect to low joint forces. Some of these ideas will be further discussed in chapter 6.

STRESS IN THE ACHILLES TENDON DUE TO PRONATION AND SUPINATION (EXAMPLE 5)

The models used in the previous examples are limited to the estimation of forces. However, the force does not describe the actual state of stress in a given anatomical structure. In order to estimate stress for the Achilles tendon, the cross-sectional area and the geometry are important, as illustrated in Figure 3.15. In order to get a feeling about the stresses in the Achilles tendon, the following simplifications are made:

1. The tendon is described as a (homogenous) band with length L, width B, and thickness D (DB = cross-sectional area).
2. The mechanical properties of the tendon are given by the stress deformation characteristics. For simplicity, we use a linear elastic model for the material.

$$\sigma\,(\Delta x) = \frac{E}{L}\,\Delta x$$

where Δx: change in length of tendon
E: modulus of elasticity

3. The bending of the tendon is described by an arc with radius R_0 (see Figure 3.16), where:

L_s: length of straight part of the tendon
L_c: length of bent part of the tendon

The length x of the tendon at the point ξ due to the bending is given by:

$$x(\xi) = (R_0 + \xi)\phi + L_s$$

The unloaded length of the tendon is:

$$x(o) = L = R_0\phi + L_s$$

The stress at the point ξ is:

$$\sigma(\Delta x[\xi]) = \frac{E}{L}\,\Delta x(\xi)$$

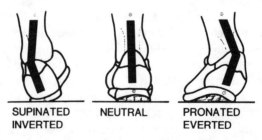

SUPINATED   NEUTRAL   PRONATED
INVERTED   EVERTED

Figure 3.15. Schematic representation of the geometry of the Achilles tendon in supinated, neutral, and pronated position. All pictures represent a left foot.

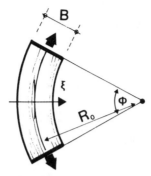

Figure 3.16. Schematic illustration of the assumptions for geometry for a tendon.

If the tension in the tendon is high enough so that the stress is positive at each point of the cross section, then the integrated stress (from $-B/2$ to $B/2$) equals

$$D \int \sigma d\xi = F = \frac{1}{L} EBDR_0 \phi$$

The stress can therefore be determined by using

$$\sigma(\xi) = \frac{F}{BD} \left(1 + \frac{\xi}{R_0}\right)$$

Example: For $R_0 = 4$ cm (corresponds to a strong pronation) and the width of the tendon $B = 2$ cm, the largest stress on the outside of the bending is about 25% higher than for a straight tendon.

COMMENTS ON EXAMPLE 5

1. Shoes do not only influence the ground reaction force but also the path of the center of pressure. Pronation and supination during stance-phase, described by the Achilles tendon angle, can be changed considerably as illustrated in Table 2.7. This emphasizes the importance of the sport shoe when considering the load on the Achilles tendon or generally on the human body.
2. An approach similar to the illustrated one may be helpful in the analysis of ligament problems. It would allow a more local analysis and, therefore, provide more specific answers.

THE STRESS IN A HINGE JOINT (EXAMPLE 6)

The pressure distribution is the relevant variable when discussing load in a joint. In order to be able to describe and/or quantify stress in a joint, the following assumptions are made (see Figure 3.17):

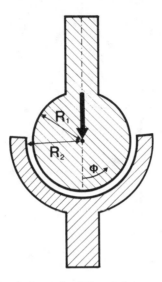

Figure 3.17. Cross-sectional view of a hinge joint.

- The bony structures are assumed to be ideally rigid.
- The geometry is determined by part of a hollow cylindrical shaft at the outside and a solid cylindrical shaft at the inside.
- Cartilage between the two surfaces is assumed to be an ideally elastic material and is described by its stress-strain characteristic (e.g., Hook).
- Effects due to ligaments are neglected and ligaments, therefore, not included.
- Cartilage is compressed under load. During compression no shear forces are generated.
- The deformation of the cartilage is small compared to the gap of the joint ($D = R_2 - R_1$).

If the relative movement of one cylinder with respect to the other one is described by the distance d, the reduction of the gap depends on the angle ϕ:

$$x(\phi) = \frac{d}{D} \cos \phi$$

Therefore the pressure is:

$$\sigma(\phi) = E \frac{d}{D} \cos \phi$$

The displacement d can be determined from:

$$\iint \sigma(\phi) \, dA = F$$

where A is the area of contact and results to:

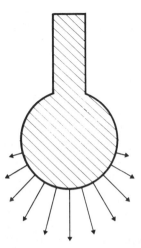

Figure 3.18. Illustration of the stress distribution in an idealized hinge joint.

$$d = \frac{2F}{\pi ELR_1} D$$

where L is the length of the cylinder.

Using this result, the stress can be determined as:

$$\sigma(\phi) = \frac{2}{\pi} \frac{F}{LR_1} \cos \phi$$

An example of such a stress distribution is illustrated in Figure 3.18. The maximal stress in a joint can therefore be estimated as:

$$\sigma_{max} = \frac{2}{\pi} \frac{F}{LR_1}$$

COMMENTS ON EXAMPLE 6

1. The example shows that the force per unit area in a joint is not constant. The maximal stress depends on the geometry of the joint. The critical limits for cartilage were determined by Yamada (1970) to 500 N/cm² for change from elastic to nonelastic and 1000 N/cm² for ultimate stress. Legal et al. (1984) published data which suggest that these limits are close to the range of everyday stresses for certain subjects. They found in a study of hip-joint disease that all analyzed subjects who had degenerative effects had stresses higher than 500 N/cm².
2. The example does not include the description of the case where the area of contact does change or where singularities in joints appear (e.g., cartilage damage). It is obvious that local stress can be a multiple of normal stress for these special cases.

SUMMARIZING COMMENTS FOR THESE EXAMPLES

The explanations and illustrations in this chapter showed that external measurements combined with modelling of the human body or parts of it can provide important knowledge which can be used to determine relevant variables in connection with running shoe analysis. The examples underline the importance of geometry in running shoe analysis. However, it is evident from the explanations that this approach is connected with difficulties, and that the development of appropriate models in connection with running shoe research (or general shoe research) is only at the beginning. The methodology for the measurement of external variables is obviously much more advanced than the development of running shoe models. Research and development of running shoes combine to make significant progress if appropriate models are available to estimate internal forces. At this time, such models are not in use in running shoe research.

Material Properties

THEORETICAL CONSIDERATIONS

When analyzing load on the locomotor system, material constants are used to describe the mechanical behavior of shoe sole, heel, and surface. The determination of those constants is usually connected with some problems and the order of magnitude of these values is not commonly known. For this reason, we have added in this chapter some methodological information, some ranges of order of magnitude of biomaterials, and some special considerations concerning the heel.

The characteristic of a shoe sole or a human heel can be described with variables usually used in material science. These variables can describe mechanical, electrical, thermic, and chemical characteristics. In connection with the load of the human body, the mechanical variables of shoe, heel, and surface are especially relevant. These variables characterize, commonly speaking, the hardness of the material, which means the resistance which is generated during deformation as a response to applied external forces. The applied force can produce tension, pressure, bending, and friction (see Figure 3.19). There exist, for example, materials which are resistant against pressure but not against friction.

Stress generated by a constant or slowly increasing force is called *static*; stress generated by a force with a high-loading rate is called *dynamic*. The response of a material to these two types of forces can be different. The resistance against deformation, which is specific for each material, is dependent on the temperature of the material, on the previous mechanical and thermic treatment, and on the shape of the material. Studies of the

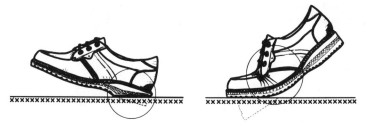

Figure 3.19. Compression and bending in a shoe.

laws of deformable materials show that the contact of two systems, for example, heel-ground, cannot be described with forces but must be described with stress. Stress is the most important term in the mechanics of deformable bodies. Deformable bodies never touch each other in isolated points like rigid bodies, rather they have a finite area of contact.

Some terms used in engineering to describe the mechanical behavior of a material are explained as follows: Normal stress (σ) with respect to an element of an area (dA) is the quotient of the force (dF) acting on this perpendicular area and the area dA

$$\sigma = \frac{dF}{dA}$$

(A general force *dF* acting obliquely on the surface area dA produces normal stress and shear stress.)

Stress and deformation are correlated in a material. A deformation requires a stress and vice versa. The real elastic or plastic behavior of a body is determined by the deformation after removing the acting forces. A body is purely *elastic* if the deformation disappears after removing the forces. A body is purely *plastic* if the deformation remains after removing the forces. This definition does not include information on the behavior of the material of interest during loading and unloading. A description of this effect is illustrated schematically in Figure 3.20. Both materials are in the above sense elastic, but they have a different behavior during dynamic loading and unloading. The two materials in Figure 3.20 are different with respect to the energy transformation. In the case on the left side, the whole energy of deformation can be transformed to mechanical work. There is no loss of mechanical energy.

In the case on the right-hand side, the loss of mechanical energy is illustrated by the dotted area. The loss of mechanical energy in itself is not a real characteristic variable of a material because it may depend on the loading rate. However, in certain cases, it is a good variable to explain differences of performance in everyday and top-level sport. The important characteristic of a material with respect to loss of energy is the dependency of the resistance on the velocity of deformation. If the stress

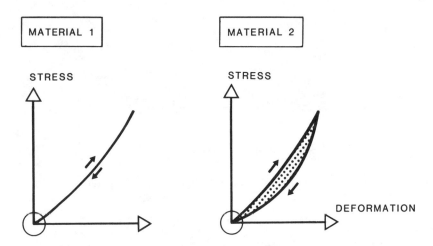

Figure 3.20. Schematic representation of two elastic materials with different mechanical behavior during deformation.

is a function of the deformation x and the velocity of deformation $\dot{x}$, the material is called viscoelastic:

$$\sigma = \sigma(x,\dot{x})$$

Each viscoelastic material transforms normally mechanical work into heat during deformation. In general, a material shows an elastic-plastic as well as a viscoelastic behavior, and the loss of energy depends on both.

MEASURING METHODS

Various methods are used to collect specific data from material. Because one dominant variable of a shoe sole and/or a playing surface is pressure, a few methods to measure the hardness of a material are described.

Shore A and D hardness test. Hardness of a material can be quantified by using an instrument which measures the resistance of a material against the penetration of a defined object under a defined pressure. The various methods applied differ mainly with respect to the form of the object. The range contains values between 0 and 100, where 0 describes the softest and 100 the hardest material. Shore A and Shore D systems based on the DIN standards are illustrated in Figure 3.21. In our measurements we consistently used Shore A values. Similar test forms were developed with an indentation hardness test (DIN 53456) where a sphere is pressed into the material of interest and a compression test (DIN 53454) where a certain pressure is applied to the material of interest.

Artificial athletes Berlin and Stuttgart. The artificial athletes, Berlin and Stuttgart (Kolitzus, 1984), are basically drop test instruments. The two

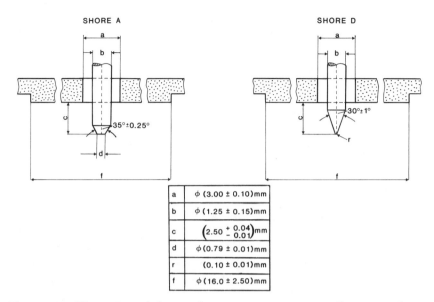

Figure 3.21. Illustration of shore value measurements using Shore A and D methods from DIN (a = 3.0 mm, b = 1.25 mm, c = 2.50 mm, d = 0.79 mm, r = 0.10 mm, f = 16.0 mm).

instruments intend to simulate the impact forces (Berlin with a dropping mass of 20 kg and a spring constant of 20 kN/cm), and the active forces (Stuttgart with a mass of 50 kg and a spring constant of 0.5 kN/cm). A similar type of drop test was used by various laboratories in modified forms (Cavanagh et al., 1980; Frederick et al., 1984). These methods commonly provide a force deformation information and a determination of the loss of energy. The artificial athletes, Berlin and Stuttgart, additionally provide a measure of the width of deflection. These methods are currently used in West Germany and some other European countries in the standards for playing surfaces. However, there is some discussion going on with respect to such standards.

MODYME—hardness. In many sport activities, surface and shoe sole can be under very high dynamic load. This was the reason for the development of various methods for impact simulation, like the artificial athlete, Berlin. Furthermore, it is important to collect information about the hardness of new and already existing surfaces in sport arenas. Based on these two demands, the MODYME (mobile dynamic measuring system) was built as explained by Nigg and Denoth (1980) and Denoth (1983).

The idea on which this measuring system is based is as follows: The stiffness of the material can be computed from the kinematics measured at touch down of a rigid body onto a material sample. The dropping mass is a rigid sphere with radius R and mass m. Touch down, deformation, rebound, and second touch down provide the necessary information for the calculation of the variables of interest. The height (H) of the free fall is variable. An accelerometer mounted on the sphere measures the acceleration and deceleration $\ddot{z}$. From the time history of acceleration the following points in time can be determined:

- beginning of free fall
- first contact of first touch down
- last contact of first touch down
- first contact of second touch down

The velocity $\dot{z}(t)$ and the displacement z(t) of the sphere for the first impact are computed by integration. The curves of acceleration, velocity, and displacement are illustrated in Figure 3.22. In this example, the history of the velocity curve shows that the sphere has a smaller velocity at take-off (last contact) after the first impact than at the first contact. Hence, the sphere lost energy during contact with the material. Furthermore, the deformation curve shows that the sphere leaves the sample when the material is still deformed. The behavior of the sample immediately after take-off of the sphere cannot be observed with this method. The reaction force F(t) is directly related to the acceleration based on the following equation

$$F(t) = m[\ddot{z}(t) + g]$$

whereby g is the acceleration due to gravity (g = 9.81 m/s²). Another way to describe the impact is the force-deformation diagram. Here the time is no longer present explicitly. The area within the curve is equivalent to the energy loss of the sphere (see Figure 3.23). Energy loss, maximum reaction force, and maximum deformation depend not only on the touch down velocity and the mass of the sphere, but also on the radius of the sphere. It makes sense, therefore, to develop a method which is independent of the testing apparatus. The goal is to achieve a stress-deformation $\sigma(z,\dot{z})$ instead of a force-deformation diagram. In order to develop such

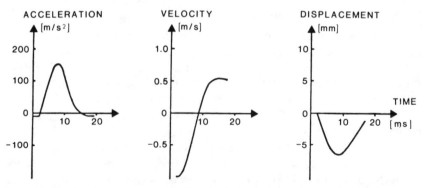

Figure 3.22. Acceleration, velocity, and displacement curves of the sphere during contact.

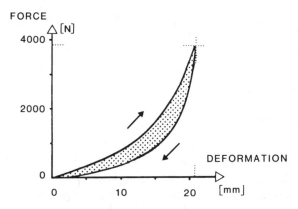

Figure 3.23. The force-deformation diagram during contact. Drop test of a sphere on a viscoelastic material.

a system, the following assumptions were made: (a) The shearing forces during deformation are small and can be neglected, which means that the material adjusts to the shape of the sphere; (b) the deformation of the material is determined by the radius of the sphere and the coordinate z at every point in time. This assumption may be replaced by a more realistic one, but the analysis will be much more complex. Using these assumptions the reaction force is related to the stress $\sigma(z,\dot{z})$ as follows:

$$F(z,\dot{z}) = 2\pi \int_0^z \sigma(z',\dot{z})[R - (z - z')]dz'$$

In the experiment, the left-hand side is known as a function of time. There are a number of mathematical possibilities to compute σ. One is to separate the ideal-elastic part from the viscoelastic part. The simplest way to describe viscoelastic behavior is a term which is proportional to velocity. This term has to be generalized under some specific conditions. For the following computations, the stress is described by the equation:

$$\sigma(z,\dot{z}) = \sigma_0(z) + a\dot{z}$$

This form of the stress demands a similar form for the force:

$$F(z,\dot{z}) = F_0(z) + 2\pi a\dot{z}z(R - 1/2z)$$

In this case, parameter "a" describes the viscoelastic behavior of the material and is therefore related to the loss of energy ΔE of the sphere. It is given by:

$$a = \Delta E/[2\pi \int_{t_0}^{t_1} \dot{z}^2(R - 1/2z)zdt]$$

The ideal-elastic part can be determined by using results from experiments. The formal connection is described by using the differential equation:

$$\sigma_0'(z) - \frac{1}{R}\sigma_0(z) = \frac{1}{2\pi R}F_0''(z), \quad \sigma_0(0) = 0$$

with $F_0(z) = [F(t) - 2\pi a\dot{z}(t)z(t)(R - 1/2z(t))](z)$

The solution of this differential equation can be expressed as a series in R. The result is:

$$\sigma_0(z) = \frac{1}{2\pi R}[F_0'(z) + \frac{1}{R}F_0(z) + \frac{1}{R^2}\int_0^z F_0 dz' + ...]$$

In this way a relatively simple description of the dynamic behavior of the material is achieved. If the assumptions are met, the force F_0 is identical during loading and unloading. Therefore F_0 is one control for how realistic the assumptions were. For small deformation z, the stress $\sigma_0(z)$ is proportional to z which seems reasonable (Hook's law). As a consequence $F_0(z)$ has to be proportional to z^2 (for small z). Should this not be the case, then the assumption "the material adjusts to the shape of the sphere" for the calculation may be wrong. The quality of this procedure is discussed in more detail by Denoth (1983). It can be summarized as follows:

1. For a touch down velocity of 1 m/s and a contact time of about 20 ms, the error of the displacement at take-off is less than 1 mm.
2. The result represents a true material information and does not depend on the testing procedure as the drop tests listed in the previous paragraphs.
3. The MODYME system can be used for measurement in various locations and does not need a laboratory set up. It can, therefore, be used to assess the quality of an installment as an example.

Examples for various tests. Figure 3.24 shows a summarized result of a drop test for 15 different surfaces currently on the market. Figure 3.25 illustrates results from a MODYME test where the data are presented in the form of a stress-deformation diagram. There is no doubt that both results can have an importance in the attempt to understand and assess such materials. The illustration in Figure 3.24 is correct and relevant for these surfaces used in 1984. Materials which will be used in 10 years may have totally different values; therefore, it is a picture of a momentary situation. The results illustrated in Figure 3.25 describe grass, a synthetic surface, and asphalt. The result that asphalt is much harder than synthetic surfaces and that out of these three, grass is the material with the smallest slope is not surprising. Much more surprising is the result: The athlete can use only about 5 mm of the synthetic surface, which had a thickness of 16 mm in this experiment. This second way of describing the material is more general and includes more information. The results illustrated in Figure 3.24 depend on the test procedure used. A dropping height of 10 cm, for instance, shows another sequence of hardness compared to a dropping height of 20 cm. Other factors influencing the results are mass

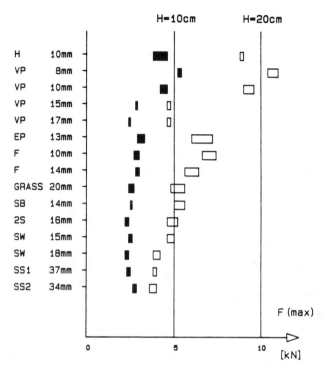

Figure 3.24. Summary of range of results from drop tests on 15 different playing surfaces. Length of bar represents the variation of three independent tests.

and radius of the sphere. The effect of the radius is illustrated in Figure 3.26. It is the result of measurements with a drop test (MODYME). The mass was kept constant. Shot 1 had a diameter of 9 cm, Shot 2 of 12 cm. The impact velocities were 1 and 2 m/s for both masses. The shore values of the materials analyzed were systematically changed from 20 to 50 shore. The materials analyzed had a thickness of 22 mm.

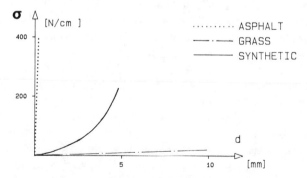

Figure 3.25. Example of a static stress-deformation diagram for asphalt, grass, and a synthetic surface.

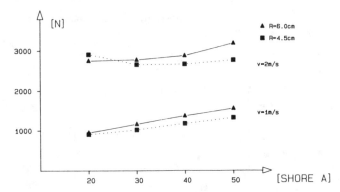

Figure 3.26. Results of MODYME hardness F_{max} versus shore hardness for two masses with different diameters but constant input energy.

The result illustrates that the shore hardness commonly used in shoe sole assessment is not the adequate hardness measure for impact studies. Area and deformation in the shore test are too small in comparison to reality. If the material is too soft, the material is totally compressed during impact and bottoms out. Therefore, the reaction force in an impact experiment at a given thickness of the material does not decrease with decreasing shore hardness, but shows a minimum for a particular shore hardness, dependent on the radius of the sphere and on the impact energy.

Mechanical Properties of Elements of the Locomotor System

In the construction of machines, the use of a large amount of material guarantees strength and reliability. If its strength is much greater than the exerted stress, the machine may be inconvenient to work with, too big, and maybe too expensive. Therefore, machines should be constructed to have a certain strength with a minimum of material. In sport activities the expressions *pain* and *injury* are very familiar, an evidence that stress exceeds critical limits. This may suggest, using the analogy of the above cited machine, that the human body is not constructed for high performance sport or that the training programs are not formed to the responses of the biomaterials of the human body, or the exerted load to strengthen the biological material.

The purpose here is to give a rough overview of some critical limits, like ultimate strength and elastic limit, and to provide some information about material properties of the human heel. It is only an overview because of three points:

Table 3.2. Order of magnitude for the modulus of elasticity, the elastic limit, and the ultimate strength for human materials (from Yamada, 1970).

Material	Modulus of elasticity (N/cm²)	Elastic limit (N/cm²)	Ultimate strength (N/cm²)	Comment
Compact bone	2,000,000	10,000	15,000	Compression
Long bone	500,000	10,000	10,000	Compression
Cartilage hyaline	50,000	500	1,000	Compression
Tendon	50,000	5,000	5,000	Tension
Ligament	500	500	500	Tension
Muscle tissue	—	—	50	Tension

1. Estimations of the stress of the different segments of the human body are at this time not very accurate.
2. In vivo measurements of ultimate strength or elastic limits are not possible, and in vitro measurements are difficult to extrapolate because the strength of biological material varies with the time between death and testing; furthermore, there exist no systematic measurements of the critical limits of subjects of different physical fitness.
3. In the last decade, a number of results on strength of biological materials were presented (Yamada, 1970; Krahl, 1976; Butler et al., 1978; Hubbard et al., 1984).

Constituent elements of the human body of interest in the context of load analysis are bone, cartilage, ligaments, tendons, and muscles. An order of magnitude of the modulus of elasticity, the elastic limit, and the ultimate strength is summarized in Table 3.2. A modulus of elasticity of 500 N/cm² means that the strain equals 2% for a compression stress of 10 N/cm². For a tibia (compressive breaking load of about 30000 N and 50 cm of length), the deformation equals 3 mm at a load of 10000 N of compression. If we assume a contact area of 10 cm² for a knee-joint, the joint force should not exceed 10000 N. In some sport activities like the long jump and gymnastics, the joint forces reach this critical value during the first impact.

The values listed above do not distinguish between static or dynamic stress or viscoelastic or plastic behavior of biological materials. The ultimate load depends on the velocity of deformation. Experimental results for a patellar tendon (Krahl, 1976) show that the ultimate force tends to be lower for slower loading rates and higher for faster loading rates. The same tendency should be true for other materials in analogy to findings from material science. This means that for an impact, the critical limits may be slightly higher than in the static or quasistatic condition.

The dominant variables which determine the load in the impact phase are the initial conditions and the hardness of the system surface-shoe-foot. In barefoot running, the hardness of the heel determines directly the magnitude of the impact peak. The mechanical properties of the heel are a meaningful information when assessing a shoe sole or a sport surface. Therefore, it is important to know the *mechanical* characteristics of the human heel. Anatomical and geometrical aspects of the heel are described extensively in text books. However, there have been no attempts to characterize the mechanical properties of the heel before 1977 (Nigg & Denoth, 1980; Cavanagh et al., 1984; Misevich & Cavanagh, 1984).

A method to measure the mechanical characteristics of the heel tissue is to estimate the hardness of the heel by an impact method (Denoth, 1981). The method used in our laboratories will be discussed in this paragraph. The test subject sits on a chair and hits the force platform with his or her heel. The lower limb moves perpendicular to the platform, so that during impact the thigh is in a horizontal position and the foot in a *dorsi-flexed* position. The online measuring variables are the reaction force F, the acceleration $\ddot{z}$ of the rigid part of the lower limb, and the impact velocity v_0. For this experimental condition, the accelerometer is mounted on top of the epicondylus lateralis. From the acceleration curve and the impact velocity the velocity-time curve and the displacement-time curve of the "rigid" part of the lower limb are calculated by integration. The displacement of the rigid part corresponds to the deformation at one point of the soft tissue and possible movements in the ankle joint.

Force-deformation diagrams for 1 subject and two different impact velocities are illustrated in Figure 3.27. It should be mentioned that in such experiments the force-time curve and the acceleration-time curve are not proportional as they are in mechanics of rigid bodies. The reason is the nonrigidness of the lower limb. The rigid mass for such impact experiments is about 50% of the mass in static cases, that is:

1. The mass of the lower limb of an adult in such experiments is about 2 kg instead of 4 kg for Δt (impact) 15 ms.

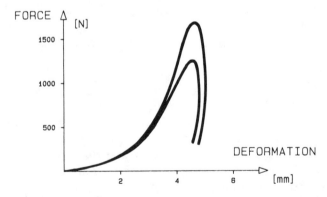

Figure 3.27. Force-deformation diagram of the heel for 1 subject (teenager) at two impact velocities.

2. If kinematic variables are used to calculate deformation, velocities, and accelerations, the relation between external (skin markers) and internal variables has to be known.

A force-deformation diagram depends on the material characteristics of the heel tissue, the geometry of the calcaneous, and the dropping mass and possible movements in the ankle joint depending on the point of application of the external force. The movement in the joint is smaller if the foot is in a dorsi-flexed position and the tibialis anterior is active. This position minimizes the maximum deformation and therefore maximizes the reaction force. The mean of the reaction force for four groups of 10 subjects at two different initial conditions and the relative deformations are shown in Figure 3.28. The four groups are defined by the age of the subjects. They are Group 1, 6-9; Group 2, 15-16; Group 3, 25-40; and Group 4, 55-80 years.

One critical point in such experiments is the first contact. From an inaccuracy of 1 ms in the first contact the deformation is influenced in the order of 1 mm at a velocity of 1 m/s. However, a shift of the force-deformation diagram of 1 mm has practically no consequence because in this flat region very little momentum is changed. In barefoot jogging, the impact velocities are generally smaller than in the experiments illustrated in Figure 3.28; the peak forces, however, are of the same order. The energy loss was estimated to be about 90% which is in agreement with the experiments of Cavanagh et al. (1984). However, he shows much more deformation of the heel (about 10 mm) at forces of about 1 times body weight. Our results cluster between 4 and 10 mm for forces between 1 and 2 times body weight. Possible reasons for this discrepancy may lie in methodological differences. One explanation may be that due to the dorsi-flexed position of the foot in our experiments, a relative movement in the joint may be reduced. Another possible explanation may be that this dorsi-flexed position exposes a more posterior aspect of the heel to the ground, and it may be that this area is harder. Recent measurements

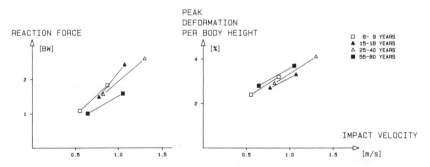

Figure 3.28. Peak reaction force (heel) relative to body weight and peak deformation relative to body height as a function of the impact velocity for four groups (n = 10, in each group).

with 1 subject during landing on the heel after a jump with ground reaction forces of about 4 times body weight resulted in deformations of only 15 mm. Because this deformation includes the movement in the joint, we speculate that the above interpretation of the difference is correct.

The geometry of the heel, which determines the contact area is very complex. The simplest approximation is a flat heel with a contact area which is constant during deformation. Then the stress-deformation diagram is proportional to the force-deformation diagram. A probably more realistic approximation is a calcaneus with the shape of a sphere. The contact area increases with increasing load. Using this assumption and a least square fit approach, as discussed in this chapter, the static stress can be described by the relation

$$\sigma_{static} \cong \frac{1}{2\pi R} \cdot \frac{dF}{dx}$$

where: F: static force
        x: deformation
        R: radius of the sphere.

The result of the analysis with 10 heels is shown in Figure 3.29. The wide range of the stress-deformation values is surprising. The human heel padding is obviously subject dependent. The reason for this wide range is not known at this time. However, this information can be used in studying the cushioning of heel-shoe and surface. The advantage of this approach lies in the fact that these results are material properties while the force-deformation results depend on the methodology of the measurement (e.g., shape of the dropping element) as illustrated by Misevich and Cavanagh (1984).

The results for the determination of the hardness of the heel can be summarized as follows:

1. The human heel becomes harder with increasing compression. In this respect, it reacts like other materials.

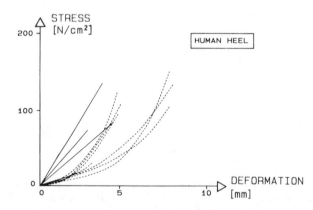

Figure 3.29. Stress-deformation diagrams for the heel of 10 subjects.

2. The most common range of heel hardness for a compression of about 5 mm is between 50 and 150 N/cm². These values are much harder than natural grass and much softer than asphalt.
3. A comparison between hardness values of shoe midsoles and heel may provide some ideas concerning selection of materials.

Influence of Movement on Load

CONTACT ELEMENT AND VELOCITY OF CONTACT

In sports activities the human body is exposed to external forces. Some of them are produced by constraints such as surface, sport equipment, or opponent. In walking, running, jogging, or jumping, the ground reaction force is the most important external force. The magnitude of the ground reaction force, its direction, and point of application have an influence on the load on the human body. Ground reaction force (magnitude and direction) and point of application depend upon several factors. Some of them will be discussed in the following.

Some general statements can be made with respect to running because this movement is periodic. The symbols used are as follows:

c = contact (time)
a = airborne (time)
cl = contact left (time)
cr = contact right (time)
cm = center of mass
k = point of application

Using these symbols, one can write for running in a straight line with constant average velocity,

vertical: $\int_{c+a} [F_z(t) - mg]dt = 0$

a-p: $\int_c F_y(t)dt = 0$

lateral: $\int_{cl} F_x(t)dt + \int_{cr} F_x(t)dt = 0$

rotation: $\int_{cl} M'(t)dt + \int_{cr} M'(t)dt = 0$

with $M' = (X_{cm} - X_k) \times F + M$

If the vertical condition is not fulfilled, the subject is running up or downhill. The anterior-posterior (a-p) condition controls the constancy of average running speed. As a matter of fact, this provides an excellent control of the experimental conditions. The lateral condition controls the straight forward running. Another aspect is the shape of the force time curves of the ground reaction forces. As illustrated in chapters 1 and 2 the impact forces are extremely shoe sensitive. During the duration of the impact peak, the following are main factors which influence impact forces:

- The contact area between surface and human body (shoe/foot)
- The geometry of the human body at this time point (joint angles)
- The state of motion of the human body and its parts (center of mass and especially contacting element)
- The material properties of surface, shoe, and heel (soft tissue)
- The preactivation of the lower extremity muscles
- The wobbling mass (Denoth et al., 1985)

The following are important factors during the active part of ground contact:

- The state of motion (cm and parts)
- The internal force generators (muscles)
- The geometry (joint angles)

This illustrates that several possibilities exist for the locomotor system to influence the shape of the ground reaction force and the moment, which means the load and stress on specific elements of the human body. Heel-strike and toe-strike are two examples of strategies in the running movement which illustrate the above mentioned possibilities. Results for internal forces for these two movement strategies are illustrated in Figure 3.30. The vertical ground reaction forces differ significantly, especially in the impact part of the ground contact. This difference is due mainly to a different contact area and contact element. The load in the lower extremities, therefore, also differs. The load in the Achilles tendon, the tibialis anterior, and the ankle joint for heel- and toe-strike is illustrated in the same figure. It was calculated using the methods illustrated in Examples 1 and 3 of chapter 2.

The purpose of this example is not the accurate determination of these forces but, once again, the basic understanding of the influence of the movement on load. The result shows that the average load in the Achilles tendon, as an example, is smaller in heel-toe running than in toe running. It also illustrates that the force in the Achilles tendon is zero during the first part of ground contact in heel-toe running. The amplitudes of the forces in the Achilles tendon during take-off are in the same order of magnitude for both types of runners. However, this result cannot be the sole basis in deciding whether one or the other style is better and should be preferred. The load distribution in the whole locomotor system in comparison with the load capacity would be one criterion on which to base such conclusions and that would be an extremely complex project! However, one can use this information in the opposite way. If an athlete has problems in the Achilles tendon, such considerations can

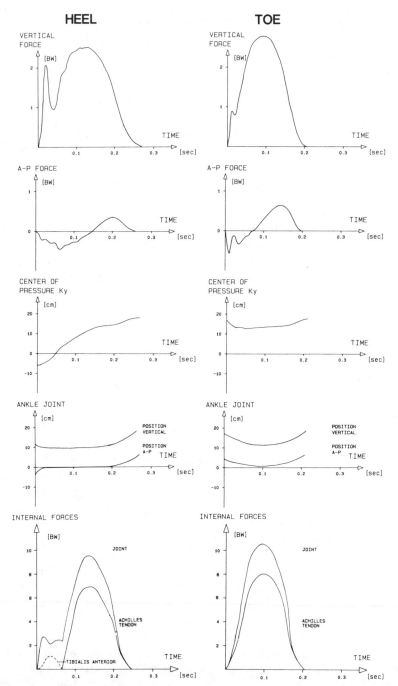

Figure 3.30. Schematic illustration of vertical and a-p ground reaction forces, center of pressure, position of the ankle joint and internal forces for heel-strike and toe-strike running ($d_{m1} = d_{m2} = 5$ cm).

be used to select the appropriate strategy. In this example, the conclusion would, therefore, be to avoid toe landing and maybe to reduce the take-off force.

As mentioned in chapter 1, the three possibilities which influence an athlete's load are movement, surface, and shoes. A smaller impact velocity reduces the magnitude of the impact peak. A softer shoe sole may have the same effect. The point of application or the path of the center of pressure is mainly determined by the way the foot contacts the ground. This, on the other hand, can be influenced by the shoe a runner is wearing. Results from studies by Nigg and co-workers (1983, 1984) showed that these movement strategies are heavily connected with the shoe. It is speculated that there is a general control strategy in humans to keep the stress below a certain level (protection mechanism). However, it is not known at this point whether this speculation corresponds to reality and, if it does, what the criteria and the applied strategies are. Figure 2.17 in chapter 2 may be the result of one of these strategies. However, because these shoes were not systematically selected, it is not possible to make a conclusion. Based on previous resarch some of the triggering influences can be listed:

- Stiffness of the surface
- Stiffness of the shoe sole
- Friction between shoe and surface
- Impact velocity of foot
- Area of contact
- Geometry (knee, rearfoot, and sole angle)

Some subjects have typical relations between some of these variables (again, see Figure 2.17), for instance, decreasing knee angle with increasing landing velocity of the heel. This aspect is not understood at all, and a general rule is not known. However, the knowledge of this aspect would be an important step forward in the understanding of running shoes and running injuries. The contact area in running is difficult to assess. One can argue that, theoretically, the total convex surface of a foot or shoe sole could be used as contact element. However, such an approach may not be satisfactory. Another way to describe the contact area is a two-dimensional strike index in analogy to Cavanagh's one-dimensional strike index (1980). This aspect has not yet found a satisfactory solution. However, experimental results illustrate how movement and, therefore, contact area as one aspect can be influenced by surface and/or shoe. Figure 3.31 shows the relative frequency of heel-strike on different surfaces for 12 subjects. The strike-index was simplified to heel-, toe-, and flat-strike. The subjects, all barefoot, were instructed to jog, to run, and to sprint a given distance. They were completely free in selecting stride length and the contact element. Impact velocity and type of contact were determined from film analysis.

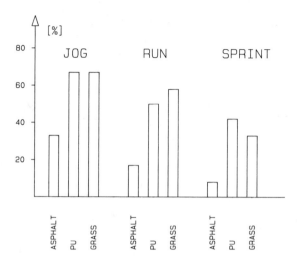

Figure 3.31. Relative frequency of heel-strike in barefoot jogging, running, and sprinting on asphalt, artificial surface (PU), and grass (averages for 12 subjects).

The results show the following:

1. The lowest frequency of heel contact with respect to surface is on asphalt in all three types of movements. Asphalt is known as being a hard surface with a medium coefficient of friction. This result is not surprising because it is common knowledge that the impact forces can easily be reduced in changing from heel- to toe-strike and running with heel-strike on asphalt may be painful.

2. The highest frequency of heel-strike is, as expected, on grass for all types of running styles. This result is probably connected with the viscoelastic properties of this surface and the relatively low impact forces on grass.

3. The result for the artificial surface (PU) is surprising. It is known that these surfaces are much harder than grass. However, the relative frequency of heel-strike is significantly higher for all running styles than on asphalt and in the same order of magnitude as on grass. This finding suggests that it may be possible that the subjective impression is used as one criterion in the selection of landing (or style) strategies. The relative frequency of occurrence of heel-strike depends, among other factors, on the running velocity. Slower jogging has consistently more heel-strike than faster running, and sprinting has the lowest percentage.

The number of subjects in this experiment is too small to make statistically significant conclusions. However, the results in connection with other observations can be used to establish the following hyotheses:

1. The softer the surface, the bigger the probability of heel-strike.
2. The slower the speed, the bigger the probability of heel-strike.

The reason for such motor behavior during running is speculated to be in the tendency of runners to control the impact loading and keep it below a certain (individual) level. Support for such an assumption can be found in acceleration measurements on the hip and the head by Nigg and co-workers (1974) and Voloshin and Wosk (1982).

If hypothesis 1 is correct, it may be expected that it would also be valid for running with shoes, although shoe and surface are not interchangeable because of the geometry aspects of a shoe. Results of an experiment with 10 subjects jogging a distance of about 1300 m in an individual, moderate velocity with two types of shoes on grass and asphalt are discussed in the following. The jogging style was not prescribed. The subjects were filmed during 10 successive steps. The results were as follows:

1. All 10 subjects chose voluntary heel as contact element on grass and asphalt with both shoes.
2. On asphalt, the impact velocity was, in general, slightly higher with the hard shoe and the knee angle bigger with the soft shoe.
3. The interindividual differences were on the average bigger than the intraindividual differences.

Both experiments show that surface and/or shoe have an influence on the running style, an influence, however, which depends very much on the individual. The second result of the second experiment appears to not be in agreement with the hypothesis because one would expect that the impact velocity for the shoe with the harder sole should be smaller compared to the values for the soft shoe. However, the increase in touch down velocity is partially corrected by a smaller knee angle for the harder shoe, which means that the effective mass is reduced. Results of recent pilot studies suggest that there are, in addition, small changes in the contact element which may have a relevant influence on the load at the ankle joint. Another possible explanation could be as follows: If the load does not exceed a certain value at the ankle joint, at tendons, or at other elements, there is from the point of view of load, no reason why a subject should change the running style. There may be other reasons for such a change such as economical aspects, force-time characteristics of the muscles, or the innervation pattern.

The theoretical considerations and the experimental results show that the shoe (and the surface) have an important influence on the running style. Support for this statement can be found in practically every chapter of this book. This change of movement pattern (style) due to shoes is connected with a change of load and stress in some elements of the runner's body. However, general rules for motor behavior strategies are not known yet, and further research is needed to investigate these relations.

NUMBER OF REPETITIONS

The influence of amount and rate of movement in sport activities is well known from a cardiovascular point of view. To be fit in jogging, an athlete may do about 10 minutes of running at a heart rate frequency of 180 minus his or her age each day, or 20 minutes at the same conditions every second day. The number of repetitions of each step or the mileage in running is an important variable in load analysis. However, little is known in this context, and for that reason, some theoretical considerations are made.

In material science, the influence of a repeated sinusoidal stress on a specific material is known. The relationship between the critical stress as a function of loading cycles is illustrated in Figure 3.32. Dead material loses its particular resistance during such a process. Dead human material may react in a similar way. However, in a living biological material, there are two aspects to be discussed in studying the effect of loading on the critical limits. One is the direct mechanical influence on the structure in analogy to dead material. The second one is the response of the biological material to the applied stress. This second response mechanism may have a positive or a negative effect on the material. In order to keep the critical limits constant, destruction and reconstruction of the material have to be in balance. If the response effect is bigger than the mechanical fatigue effect, the tissue is strengthened. It is known that cartilage and tendon material show little response to a stimulus because of a low nutrition flow. Bone and muscles, however, show a much higher response. In order to estimate biopositive or bionegative effects of running activities, one should know more about the material properties of biomaterials. However, this aspect of repetitive loading and fatigue problems in running is only in a very rudimentary stage of development.

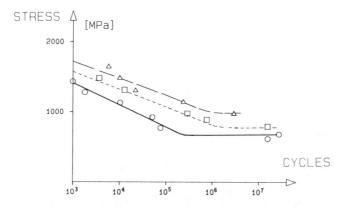

Figure 3.32. Relationship between critical stress and number of loading cycles for stainless steel.

FORCES IN JOINTS AND LIGAMENTS DEPENDING ON MOVEMENT

In a simplified locomotor system, a joint consists of a cartilaginous surface and ligaments. Acting forces produce pressure on cartilage and tension on ligaments. The acting force can be an impact force or a force with a slowly changing loading rate such as the ground reaction force during the active phase in jogging. The force in the joint and (possible) influences of the shoe will be illustrated with the example heel-strike. A schematic shape of the ground reaction force is shown in various figures of this book. A simple model to describe the impact peak in the force-time curve is described in chapter 3 (Example 3). This 3-link model (without muscles and without foot) results in the relation for the vertical component of the force acting at the knee joint:

$$F_{impact\ j} = [(m^* - m_1)/m^*]F_{impact\ e}$$

The factor $(m^* - m_1)/m^*$ as a function of the knee angle is illustrated in Figure 3.33.

If the ground reaction force and the knee angle are known, the force in the knee joint can be estimated. During jogging, the knee angle is between 155° and 175°. Therefore, the impact peak at the knee joint is about 70% of the peak at the ground which is about 1.6 times body weight. Thus, the peak at the knee joint is about 1.4 to 2.1 times body weight. This peak can be influenced by a shoe in a direct or in an indirect way. The hardness of a shoe sole, as well as the geometry and stiffness of the sole, have a direct influence. An indirect influence of the shoe is produced by changes of the running style. For example, a smaller impact velocity, consequently, has a smaller force peak. Changing the knee angle means

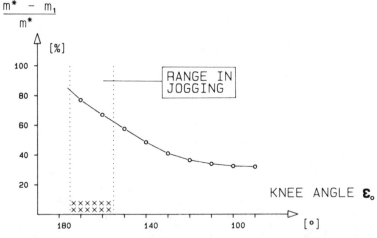

Figure 3.33. Influence of the knee angle on the ratio $(m^* - m_1)/m^*$.

changing the effective mass. Therefore, the force peak is changed, too. Changing the way of the touch down (for example, from a touch down at the lateral part of the heel to the middle part) has as a consequence a different contact area and different lever arms at the point of application with respect to the ankle joint.

The force in the knee joint during the active phase of the movement can be estimated quasistatically. In the most simplified case, it leads to an estimation of the lever arms with respect to the knee joint (Figure 3.34). d_e is the distance between ground reaction force F_e and joint, d_m the distance between a (single) muscle force F_m and the joint. In the quasistatic case the relation holds:

$$F_e d_e \sim F_m d_m$$

In most cases, the muscle force F_m may exceed the ground reaction force by a factor of 4, because the quotient d_e/d_m determines the muscle force.

A rough estimation of the joint force is given by:

$$F_{active\ j} \cong \frac{d_e + d_m}{d_m} F_{active\ e}$$

For a distance $d_e = 12$ cm and $d_m = 4$ cm, the joint force is 4 times the ground reaction force. The joint force during the active phase is not directly influenced by the hardness of the shoe sole. However, the geometry of the shoe sole, the running style, and the innervation pattern influence the force in the knee joint. The maximum force at the knee joint is larger in amplitude than the peak force during the active phase.

With respect to stress, the impact and active phase differ in the variable time. The importance of this variable is discussed in a hypothetical example of a loose joint. A gap between the two cartilaginous surfaces, as a consequence, for example, of strained ligaments and/or a wrong innervation pattern, behaves differently during the impact and active phase. In the active phase, the joint force increases slowly and the surfaces have

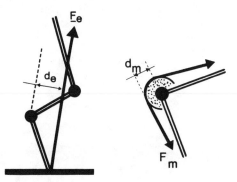

Figure 3.34. Schematic representation of the lever arms in a knee joint (lateral view).

enough time to move in an ideal position. However, in the impact phase, the two surfaces collide. As a consequence, the peak pressure in the impact phase may easily exceed the peak pressure in the active phase.

An additional comment should be made with respect to ligaments. A ligament is a passive element in comparison to the muscle, the force generator. It behaves like a viscoelastic material. Such a material can be characterized (depending on the problem to be solved) by a set of parameters. The stress in a ligament is described in a simple model by the strain and its velocity. Both can be estimated by kinematic variables such as angles, angular velocities, and lever arms. The force in a muscle, however, depends on the active state of the muscle. Therefore, the behavior of a muscle on an external force differs from the behavior of a ligament. The ligament reacts in a completely determined way. The reaction of a muscle, however, depends on its activation. If the muscles are not active, they will stretch "without" resistance. For higher activation, the resistance increases and the strain decreases. Because of a time delay between innervation and force-production, the nervous control system has to act *before* the external force acts. Therefore, a muscle may only replace the function of a ligament if the force strain characteristic is the same with respect to the joint as the characteristic of the ligament. This is only possible for slow movements which we describe as active phase and not for the impact phase.

4

ALEX STACOFF
SIMON M. LUETHI

Special aspects of shoe construction and foot anatomy

The first chapters explain the general justification to study load on the locomotor system in connection with running and running shoes. It has been shown that two out of three runners are injured once per year which indicates that the locomotor system was overloaded. In chapters 2 and 3, experimental and theoretical possibilities to quantify load in connection with running and running shoes are discussed. The measurement of external variables was the approach commonly used in the past. However, it seems evident that internal forces are of interest. In order to calculate internal variables, information about the orientation of joints and lever-arms is needed. It is evident that these calculations must be based on the knowledge of the anatomy of both the shoe and foot. Some of these anatomical aspects of general or specific interest in this context are briefly discussed in this chapter. The main purpose is to give an overview and to provide the reader with perspectives. More detailed discussions of several of these aspects, especially of foot anatomy, can easily be found in textbooks.

The first part of this chapter describes the various parts of a running shoe. Special attention is given to the last and the inserts. The second part discusses anatomical aspects of the foot. Each part is subdivided in an external typology and an internal description with special emphasis on pronation and supination. Some attempts are made to apply some of the anatomical information to the shoe in a general and systematic way.

Shoe Construction

A running shoe is constructed out of 15-20 individual parts or construction elements which are stitched and cemented together in a very specific way. The making of a shoe is a handicraft which still has room for good to bad quality in the end-product. Given two assembly lines, one with experienced shoemakers and one with novices, two very different shoes may come out, even though the same materials, tools, and machines were used. Good shoemakers know when they have made good shoes because they have developed their own standards. Experience tells them how to handle different types of material and what tricks they can use for the best outcome. However, on the assembly line, shortcuts and compromises often have to be made for practical and economical reasons. Compromising can happen, in particular, on a shoe of the lower price range in which some elements are simply left out in the final shoe construction. From experience (i.e., feedback from the customers) shoe manufacturers seem to know which parts of a shoe are important and which can safely be left out.

When making prototypes of newly designed shoes, however, it is much more difficult to judge the effect of one construction element on the runner and his or her performance. Runners are very sensitive to relatively small changes in the shoes. It has probably happened to almost any dedicated runner that "something didn't feel the same in the left shoe when compared to the right." By carefully comparing the shoes, the runner may have found small, but crucial differences, such as a different alignment of the heel counter, an insert or support not put in the same place in the two shoes, or a differing stiffness of the sole material. The hardy runner normally accepts this as part of the variance with which shoes are produced, and after a few more miles he or she may get used to it, and the shoe is "broken in." Note, too, that the runner may well have two different (asymmetrical) feet and may never have realized that.

Figure 4.1 illustrates various elements of a running shoe. Some of these construction elements have been altered and changed to different forms and shapes by the shoe industry over the last few years. Changing the design of an article offers two advantages: It may be that the quality of the product is improved, or that the product changes in appearance and looks new. But how can one know whether a new shoe element is really an improvement or just a gimmick? When trying to find out whether or not a new shoe element works, the shoe industry can use the traditional trial and error method, combined with a large body of experience of what works and what does not. Surely, some great shoes have been put on the market in this manner, but some runners probably suffered injuries due to the errors along the way. However, when shoe researchers want

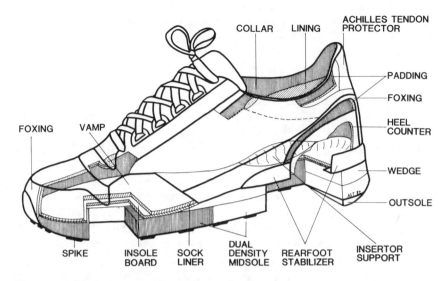

Figure 4.1. Various parts of a running shoe.

to understand the effect of one shoe element, they usually do not apply the trial-and-error method. Special test shoes are designed in which one construction element is altered systematically. Thus, if one wants to find the effect of the length of heel counters, one has to study about five different heel counters, ranging from short to long, on running shoes which are otherwise exactly the same. However, if 20 shoe elements are varied over a range of five systematic steps, it adds up to the large number of 95,367,431,640,625 test shoes. Clearly, this is too time-consuming to test. Therefore, priorities have to be specified. From the many elements that form a shoe, very few have been subjects of a systematic analysis. In fact, the insert in the shoes and the midsole material are the main elements of shoe construction which have been examined somewhat closely.

HISTORICAL DEVELOPMENT OF THE LAST

The centerpiece of the shoe, the last, draws relatively little attention. This may be due to the complexity of the problems involved or to the fact that the development of the shoe lasts lies almost entirely in the hands of companies who do not like to share their experiences with others too openly.

The word *last* originates from Old English *laesk*, which means sole, footprint, or track. The first lasts were chiselled out of stone, and later, whittled out of wood. In the early 19th century, the machine for shaping gunstocks was converted to become a last-turning lathe (Rossi, 1980). Thus, it was possible to form a last with a machine, and the first last-making plant with lathes was established in Lynn, Massachusetts, in 1820. In 1969, the plastic last was developed by the Sterling Last Corporation, U.S.A. In contrast to wood, the plastic last does not stretch or swell with changes in temperature or humidity. Today, the shoe industry is mostly using plastic lasts.

The form of the last has been a reason for complaints for centuries. The Greeks (i.e., Paul of Sagina) described injuries which came from wearing shoes. Camper complained in 1783 that the same lasts were used for right and left shoes and hoped that his "mockery would help to improve the shoes." But the same "straight" lasts (there was no left and right) were used until the end of the 19th century. It took Hermann von Meyer's devoted intervention. To change the situation, in 1860 he wrote in his book *Die richtige Gestalt der Schuhe* (*The Right Form of the Shoes*) that "most people suffer from badly constructed shoes." Von Meyer found "fashion detrimental on the mechanism of the foot," a statement which is still surely true today. The correct form of the last, according to von Meyer, was such that the line which was drawn parallel to the toeline passed through the center P of the heel. When the line did not pass through point P, the shoe was criticized by von Meyer. This applies for shoes today, as well (Figure 4.2).

Von Meyer's shoes looked inflared or curved in comparison to the straight lasts that were used at that time. This started an argument about straight or curved lasts which still continues today, although today's straight last has nothing to do with the straight last of the 19th century. When aligning the rearfoot of different running shoes (Cavanagh, 1980),

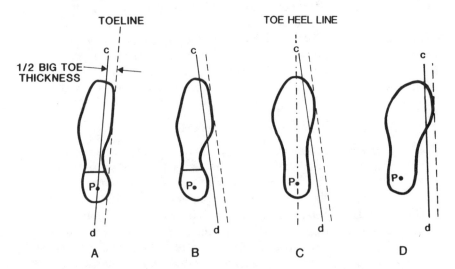

Figure 4.2. Tracings from the last bottom papers. (A) Correct curved form after von Meyer. (B) Incorrect straight form after von Meyer. (C) Today's straight running shoe form. (D) Today's curved running shoe form.

even today's straight last looks curved. However, when connecting the two ends of the shoe sole with a line (toe-to-heel line), today's straight last "looks actually straight." Cavanagh (1980) suggested that the difficulty of explaining these curved or straight shoes lies in "that the footprint resembles an inflared shoe, while the foot outline resembles a straight one." For curiosity's sake, one might consider von Meyer's standard (the c-d line passing through P) on today's shoes and find that probably none of these shoes would pass. The discussion about straight or curved lasts will probably continue as long as different measuring techniques are used.

A running shoe must fit not only in overall length and ball width, but with respect to several other aspects such as the instep, arch, top lines, and heel and toe curve. Each of these can be measured, but vary depending on the type of footwear, for example, jogging shoes, racing flats, fashionable shoes, and so on. The complexities of adjustments are very large, and it is not surprising that only a few last model makers are known in each country. In the U.S., for instance, there are probably not more than 25 last model makers in the whole industry (Rossi, 1980). Various small but important features are built into a last, for example, the toe spring and heel spring. The toe spring (often around 5 mm) allows a slight rocking effect during take-off. It has to be carefully calculated, but in general, the higher the heel or the thicker the midsole, the more toe spring is required.

Heel spring became more important because sport shoe companies decided to increase heel height for better shock absorption of the shoes using the same shoe lasts. Now the runners started to slide forward in the shoes which created problems on the toes (blisters, black nails). When raising the heel, a new last should be created in order to avoid these problems as illustrated in Figure 4.3. The new last has to be changed in several parts: The heel spring (now higher) requires the pitch to be changed and the toe spring to be adapted. But also the back of the last has to allow more room for the heel. Now, the shoe fits the runner comfortably again without hurting the toes.

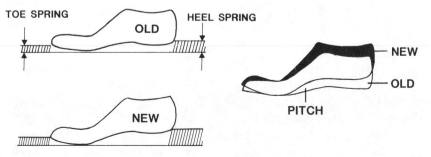

Figure 4.3. Heel and toe spring with increased heel height.

INSERTS

A large variety of elements which have various names, such as inserts, arch supports, arch cookies, orthotics, and orthoses, can be put into a shoe. For the sake of consistency, the expression *insert* was chosen to be used in this review. An insert can be of any form and size; all it requires is that it can be put or glued into a shoe.

The history of shoe inserts goes back to the 18th century when Petrus Camper (professor in Franeker, Friesland) constructed the first insert from cork material. This was the start of an evolution throughout the next 2 centuries where a large number of inserts were developed from traditional materials such as leather, cork, wood, and different metals. Most of the early developers were from Germany, where this topic attracted over 30 authors until the middle of the 20th century.

An exception was Whitman who in 1887 constructed an insert which is still well known in the U.S. Whitman's insert had a high rim on the medial and lateral side and was formed from sheet copper. Like almost all other inserts, it was constructed with the help of a negative and positive cast and with plaster of paris. In preparation of this form, the patient was usually in a sitting position while a possible foot deformity was corrected. With the help of the cast, Whitman constructed inserts which, in the view of other podiatrists, caused problems to the user, particularly in the arch region of the midfoot where the insert came out with too high an arch (Massart, 1938). This was first recognized by Lange (1914) who had the patient putting down part of his body weight during the formation of the plaster form. Lange also introduced a new material, celluloid, which he combined with steel bands to a very sophisticated insert. Lange's insert was modified by several authors during the first 2 decades of this century.

The family Berkemann is often given credit for the first industrially produced insert in 1905, although Riker in 1901 (from Cavanagh, 1980) and Wagner in 1899 are known to have had their products appear on the market a few years earlier. These inserts had the advantage that they did not need any plaster form and could simply be laid into the shoe. This technique was certainly cheaper than the handmade inserts with the plaster construction, but they were not individually adapted for each patient.

Today, both constructions of inserts are well in use, the industrially produced insert for the over-the-counter market, and the plaster construction often for more severe orthopaedic problems. Another conventional type of insert was put out in 1924 by Dr. Scholl, whose inserts are still widely distributed. The same is to be said about Mau's insert in 1933, used mostly by women, and Blount's insert in 1931, which are widely distributed in the U.S. On the material side, the revolution started in the late 1930s when Plexidur and later different plastics came into use.

With the first edition of *Orthopaedie des Fusses,* Rabl (1944) established a fundamental work for orthopaedic surgeons and orthopaedic shoemakers with many practical hints for both fields. Rabl mentions that the position of the medial insert should be based on experience at the highest point, around one-fourth from the back of the foot. This should be applied with some caution because the calcaneus varies quite extensively among different subjects. Zamosky (1964) reported on a "cookie insert" and a navicular pad whose highest points were positioned in the area of the talonavicular joint at the medial side. These shoe modifications, the latter one being softer than the former, were proposed for restoring foot balance in standing and walking. The different opinions about the position of the medial insert clearly show that personal experience and not well-defined experiments dictate the decision making of where the foot should be supported in a shoe.

Inserts in the running shoe. Since the running boom started in the early 1970s, in particular in North America, a new sport shoe insert market developed right along with it. The old types of inserts, traditionally used in hospitals or by podiatrists, consist even now of leather, cork, wood, and metals. The inserts for the sport shoe market consist of many different types of plastics and E.V.A. (Ethylene Vinyl Acetate). The market offers quite a variety of inserts, particularly for joggers and runners. Recently, inserts were developed which mold with a thermoplastic technique to the subject's feet.

Another type of insert is the built-in insert which is incorporated into or onto the sole of the shoe. This is a rather rare form of conventional shoe construction. However, there are a few patents available which are not realized on the market. Bierregaard (1945) constructed a shoe insert for flatfeet consisting of wedges under the forefoot and rearfoot which were tilted on opposite sides (Figure 4.4). In this way, the anatomical stability of the overcivilized foot was said to be regained. Hayward (1975) handed in a patent for an orthopaedic canvas shoe containing a "supporting arch." The new idea was to position the insert in such a way that

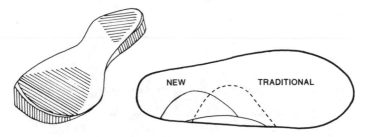

Figure 4.4. Inserts by Hayward (1975) on the right and Bierregaard (1945) on the left side.

its highest point came under the navicular point rather than further forward as often used in sport shoes (Figure 3.33). However, this was already proposed by Rabl (1944) and Zamosky (1964), but was probably not registered as a patent in the U.S. It is interesting that this strategy corresponds to results summarized in chapter 6. Adidas France (1977) claimed a patent which lifted the medial border of the foot all along the length of the shoe. This varus wedge idea goes back to the 1930s (according to Cavanagh, 1980) when it was used in basketball shoes and later (1958) in army boots. For running shoes, it was put on the market by Brooks Inc., who present several shoes with this feature. The reasoning supporting this shoe construction is that it would help to reduce pronation and injuries that go with it.

Whatever positive effects shoe inserts can have, one aspect has to be looked at carefully: Shoe inserts should not raise the heel within the shoe so that the shoe cannot support the foot against pronation. Most running shoes grasp and hold the foot with a heel cap of 5 to 7 cm in height. Shoe inserts can easily make up 1 to 1.5 cm in height, which raises the heel within the shoe considerably (Figure 4.5).

Putting inserts into a running shoe leads to another critical aspect. Due to the higher position of the heel the axes of rotation are moved upward, which may influence the lever arms for the acting forces. The result may, therefore, be a change in the acting moments or an adaptation of the foot movement. Using such an insert, one has to be aware of the possible positive or negative aspects induced. Whenever the geometry (in this case the height of the joint axes) is changed, the transfer of external to internal forces is changed as illustrated in chapter 3, and it must be studied carefully.

Effects of an insert. Many authors who write about inserts are quite positive about one thing: Inserts do something to the runner's foot. However, exactly what it is they do is not altogether clear. Surely, there

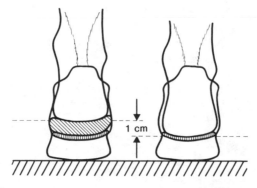

Figure 4.5. Different geometric situation with (left) and without (right) an insert at the heel.

exist a broad variety of inserts, different views of looking at one particular problem (i.e., injuries), and a large number of feet and running styles. There are a few authors, however, who have published on the actual effects of inserts, particularly the effects during the support phase of a running stride.

Among the first to describe the effects of inserts in running shoes was Subotnick (1979, 1981) who stated that an insert would

> Merely allow the foot to get into the proper position so that the muscles can do their job in aligning the joints, and the bony architecture of the foot can do its job in actually supporting the body weight.

Subotnick's patients receive two types of inserts, the *rigid* or *functional* inserts, which are used every day and for long-distance training, and the *flexible* inserts, which are utilized in sprinting, field-events, and different ball games. The flexible insert is also used for preparing the athlete for more rigid inserts. Both types, however, are based on the making of a cast of the foot "as it is held in the nonweight bearing neutral position" when the patient lies in a prone position on the examination table. The prescription of an insert follows when the foot needs to be stabilized around this neutral position. Such neutral orthoses (inserts) are assumed to prevent compensation and to maintain the foot in its individual neutral position, a procedure which is widely accepted by podiatrists in North America. A forefoot varus is, therefore, supported by an insert on the medial side of the forefoot which provides contact of the whole forefoot with the ground without changing the neutral position of the rearfoot. Therefore, this strategy does not correct (change) the forefoot position (Figure 4.6, left). A rearfoot valgus is often counterbalanced with an insert on the medial side, helping to prevent excessive pronation (Cavanagh, 1980) as illustrated in Figure 4.6, center. This could be considered as a *corrective* type of insert in contrast to the forefoot varus wedge which is supporting the individual's neutral position.

Effects of inserts during the contact phase of a runner's foot were first described by Nigg et al. (1977) and Nigg et al. (1978) using film analysis.

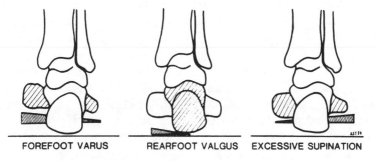

FOREFOOT VARUS   REARFOOT VALGUS   EXCESSIVE SUPINATION

Figure 4.6. Examples of inserts for special foot types.

Some of the conclusions were that a good insert should change the gait characteristics toward the values hypothesized to be characteristic of healthy feet. Their results suggested that for good medial support, the insert should be placed further back in the shoe under the sustentaculum tali of the calcaneus as discussed in chapter 6. The forefoot insert against excessive supination was found to be most effective at the lateral side of the forefoot (Figure 4.6, right), which is the opposite correction to the one for the forefoot varus. This may also be considered as a corrective type of insert.

Bates et al. (1979) studied pronation during the support phase of 6 runners. The subjects repeated the trials barefoot, and in shoes with and without inserts. The subjects pronated most running barefoot, which is in contrast to the findings reported by Nigg and Luethi (1980) who noted that least pronation occurred in the barefoot condition. Both authors agree, however, that it is possible to ''modify the lower extremity mechanics of injured runners in such a way that the observed values were similar to those measured on uninjured runners wearing a simple shoe and no insert.'' Cavanagh (1978) investigated the effect of increased thickness of the inserts put on the medial side of the shoe and found reduction of pronation with increasing thickness.

The value of inserts. In conclusion, the often noted question, ''Do inserts work?'' can be answered with a differentiated ''yes'': a ''positive yes'' because the effects of the inserts on the runners' running style can be shown with biomechanical methods, and because various clinics (Subotnick, 1979; Clement, 1982; Segesser et al., 1982) report a success rate of 70-90% when applying inserts to runners; a ''negative yes'' because different schools of applying inserts seem to have equal success despite the fact that their inserts look quite different. The description of the state of the art of running shoe inserts shows that the development was mainly based on experience. Note that this is not a negative comment. However, it is assumed that new developments should be based on reflections and considerations discussed in various chapters of this book.

In the future, the podiatrist may work together with the biomechanists—a joint relationship which may appear as follows:

1. A patient visits the medical specialist because of a running injury.
2. The medical specialist diagnoses the injury and defines the anatomical location (tendon, ligament, etc.) where the overload takes place.
3. A biomechanic specialist analyzes various strategies which can be used to reduce load in this structure and checks the influence of such a strategy on other structures involved. Based on this analysis, he proposes several possibilities which could be used to solve the problem.
4. The medical specialist decides upon the strategy to use based on this information.

It is evident that such a procedure has to be on line and cannot take days or weeks. Furthermore, the decision has to be based on a dynamic assessment. It would be advantageous if the effect of different strategies could be assessed on site, and if the selected solution could be controlled after a short time (maybe 2 weeks).

OTHER SHOE CONSTRUCTION CONCERNS

The explanations in the last few pages may produce the impression that last and insert are the two main aspects in the construction of a running shoe, and that these are the two main elements that influence and control impact, pronation, and supination. This is, of course, not the case. Last and insert were used to demonstrate the historical development because these elements were used for decades or even centuries in shoe construction. However, in the last 10 to 20 years, many new ideas were developed in running shoe construction and applied to reduce impact forces and/or to reduce pronation or supination. It is of general interest to understand the possibilities of these construction strategies.

In the following, a discussion of some of these elements is presented. From our point of view, the most important question is if and how the transfer function between external and internal forces is influenced. Some of the changes may influence the lever arms between acting forces and joints, which were described as a change in geometry. This significantly influences the transfer function between external and internal force. Some other changes may influence the magnitude of the forces without significantly changing the lever arms, which usually is produced by a change in material. This would *not* change the transfer function between external and internal force. Obviously, these two aspects are correlated and we think it is necessary to determine the main effect of any change on the internal loading.

Some theoretical examples may illustrate this idea. One element which is widely varied in shoe construction is the midsole. It is constructed differently in geometrical form and material properties. One geometrical solution is the flare at the lateral part of the heel. A variation of this lateral heel flare from $30°$ to $-30°$ produces, primarily, a shift of the line of action of the ground reaction force toward the joint. The lever arm is reduced. This change of flare, therefore, has two main effects: The external impact forces are increased and the moment of rotation in the subtalar joint, responsible for the pronation, is decreased. One can, therefore, expect an increase in the externally measured impact force and a decrease in the externally measured pronation velocity.

Another theoretical example is the change of hardness of the midsole with constant flare (e.g., $15°$). Such a change would again produce two main effects: The deformation of the material would increase for softer materials if it does not bottom out; and, additionally, the line of action would move toward the joint, which would reduce the lever arm. The first effect would produce a decrease in the external and internal impact force. However, the second effect would increase these impact forces again. The result could therefore be that the expected change in impact forces would not occur (Kaelin et al., 1984), but as a side effect, pronation could be reduced.

These examples clearly illustrate that changes in the midsole may influence geometry as well as deformation. Deformation has some connection with cushioning as explained in chapter 3. Furthermore, they show that shoe sole geometry and deformation may often be connected. Finally, they suggest that the results of pronation and cushioning one wants to produce can be achieved by a change of geometry and/or material of the midsole. However, these examples also show that one may well produce unwanted side effects if changes due to shoe construction are not carefully controlled.

Changes in midsole geometry and material are only one of various strategies which can be used to alter the properties of a running shoe. Heel counters, heel stabilizers, insoles, inserts, additional wedges, and different lasts are some additional strategies used in running shoe construction. Many of them are used in combination with others which may introduce additional problems in quantifying their effects. There is no unique solution. All have advantages which can be used and disadvantages that have to be dealt with. The crucial consideration is their influence on the geometry and deformation of foot and shoe. Each comprehensive approach must take into consideration both of these aspects. Impact tests currently used analyze only the second aspect. They, therefore, have limited relevance as long as they are not completed by information on shoe and foot geometry.

Anatomy of the Foot

One approach when studying the foot is from the outside, describing the various shapes of a foot which would result in a typology. Another possibility is to discuss the inside, including the various anatomical elements, their functions, their geometrical alignment, and their material properties. In this chapter, first, the typology and then the inside aspects will be discussed.

When trying to achieve outstanding results in running, a large number of factors may influence the total effort. One of these factors is certainly the geometry or physique of an athlete's body. Generally, there are some trends that can be recognized among coaches and trainers that may sound like this: "For a long distance runner you have got to be . . ." The description is usually subjective and often depends on personal experience. A more objective way of describing body composition is *somatotyping*, a method which includes body weight, height, and fat and muscle girth in the overall picture. The method originates from Sheldon and was later improved by several authors. In sport circles, it was used by Tanner who reported data from the Commonwealth Games 1958 and the Olympic Games 1960 (Tanner, 1964). Among runners, Tanner was able to distinguish most athletes, such as sprinters, middle, and long distance runners. Exceptions, however, were noted, because the two Olympic winners Snell (800 m, 1500 m) and Berruti (200 m) did not fit into the categories in which they were thought to belong.

When trying to categorize the geometry of the feet, similar problems arise. What does the typical foot of a marathoner look like? Should a sprinter have a flat foot or a high arched one? Several attempts were made in the past to categorize feet with respect to form and/or function. Feet can be classified by their external appearance in different types. Examples of such classifications are shown in Figure 4.7 based on work by Debrunner (1982). The *normal* foot, which is also called the *unobtrusive foot*, is characterized by an arch of medium height, by a straight impression of the footprint (*podogram*), and by a vertically aligned rearfoot. The *flatfoot* (pes planus) is characterized by a low arch (or no arch at all) which can be illustrated with a wide podogram in the midfoot region. Sometimes the footprint gives the impression that the foot is toeing-out (abducted). It is frequently in a valgus position. The *high arch foot* (pes cavus) is characterized by its high arch which results in a footprint limited just to the forefoot and rearfoot. High arch feet are sometimes connected with valgus or with varus positions, particularly when the rearfoot stability is weak. (Note that there exists also the *splayfoot* which appears frequently with high arch feet. The forefoot is relatively wide and pressure may appear in the footprint under the bases of the second and third toe [pes transversus].)

As in somatotyping this external description does not take into account what the athlete is actually doing with his or her foot during performance. Some orthopedic surgeons are very critical when looking at the traditional ways of examining feet. Segesser (1980), for example, states that "no well-founded statements of prophylactic value can be made about the dynamic capacity of a foot from present clinical methods of orthopedic examination" (translation by the author). Hlavac (1977) concluded that

> In the past, specific abnormalities were noticed in the resting position, certain things were noticed in the standing foot and other major neuromuscular deformities were noticed in gait. Therefore, treatment of these problems was empirical and did not relate to an understanding of function.

What is needed in particular for the evaluation of feet of athletes is a categorization of feet during performance. Clarke (1980) went in this direction when grouping feet of similar distribution of pressure, which corre-

FOOTTYPE	HEIGHT OF LONGITUDINAL ARCH	REARFOOT POSITION	PODOGRAM
NORMAL	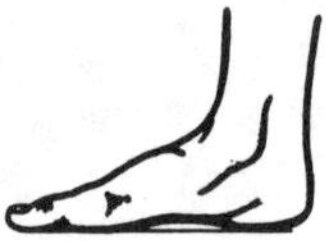	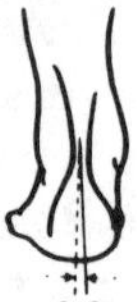 0–6°	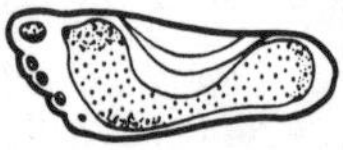
PES PLANUS	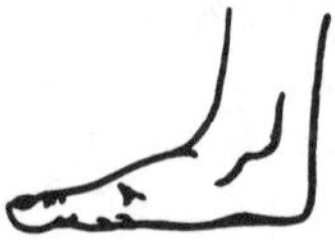		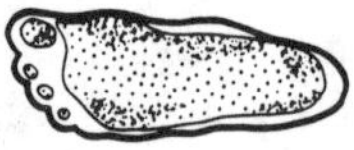
PES CAVUS	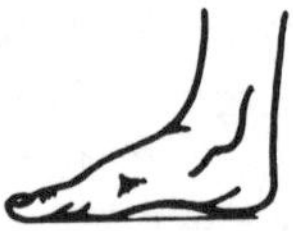		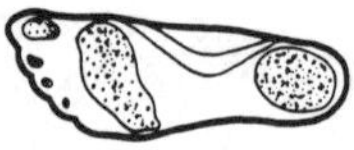
PES VALGUS		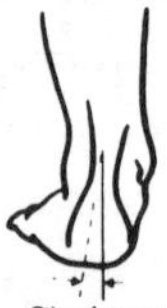 6° and more	
PES VARUS		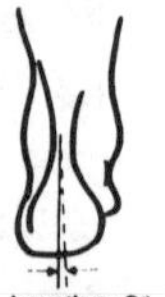 less than 0°	

Figure 4.7. Possible categorizations of feet based on Debrunner (1982).

lated with the clinicians classification, by a correlation coefficient of $r = 0.75$. However, more effort is needed before function of the feet during performance is clearly understood and can be categorized. The following pages are an attempt to describe the human foot from a mechanical-anatomical point of view. Important elements such as bones, joints, ligaments, muscles, and tendons are discussed briefly with a description of their dynamic function, and some order of magnitude of forces and their lever-arms.

The complex skeletal system of the foot is composed of 26 bones which can be divided into three segments: tarsus, metatarsus, and the phalanges. The 26 bones consist of 7 tarsals, 5 metatarsals, and 14 phalangeal bones (see Figure 4.8). The posterior part (tarsus) comprises the talus located at the apex of the foot and the calcaneus (heel bone) which forms the hindmost portion of the foot and contacts the ground first during heel-strike in running. Both bones are so-called short bones and are irregular in shape. During running (heel-strike), these two bones are exposed to impact forces at initial contact. The forces are transmitted through them to the upper parts of the lower extremities. Talus and calcaneus are connected by a freely movable joint system, the subtalar joint. Furthermore, both bones articulate with other tarsal bones and the talus, together with the shank, forms the ankle joint.

The other five tarsal bones (navicular, cuboid, and the three cuneiforms) are located anteriorly to the talus and calcaneus and together form a structure which is often called the midfoot. Although they are movable against each other, the range of motion of these small joints is very restricted mainly because of a number of ligaments which hold the structure tightly together. However, it should be noted that the midfoot is not a rigid construction. In a normal foot, these bones usually do not make contact with the ground during walking or running. The metatarsus or forefoot consists of five short long bones, the metatarsals. Their proximal bases articulate with each other as well as with the tarsus and hence usually are off ground, whereas the distal bases contact the ground during stance

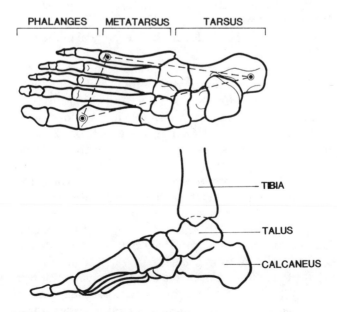

Figure 4.8. The skeletal structure of the foot.

phase and push-off. The metatarsals serve mainly to resist compressional load, similar to other long bones in the body (e.g., tibia, femur).

The toes consist of 14 bones (phalanges), the same number of bones found in a hand. The big toe (hallux) has two large phalanges. The other four toes have three smaller phalanges. Although in some books, the toes are referred to as being "leftovers" of evolution, they certainly have to fulfill special tasks, especially when the rearfoot is off ground (e.g., second part of the stance phase in running).

During standing, the foot is mainly supported at three points: the calcaneus and the distal bases of the first and fifth metatarsals (Figure 4.8). This is a result of the way bones are arranged within the foot forming the arches of the foot. One can distinguish between a longitudinal arch and a transverse arch. The medial aspect of the longitudinal arch is higher than the lateral aspect. On the load-bearing foot, these arches tend to be flattened. Certain structures counteract against this tendency in order to maintain the arches. Overloading of these structures during running can result in more or less severe pain (e.g., strain of plantar ligaments).

The major joints in the foot are synovial joints. They consist of at least two articulating bones, a joint cavity, and a space between the bones. A synovial joint is embedded in a joint capsule, which consists of several layers and a small amount of synovial fluid on the inside. Synovial joints are also characterized by the presence of articular cartilage, a thin gel-like layer which minimizes friction between the two bones and acts in a limited way as a shock-absorbing structure. In some synovial joints, small articular discs (menisci in the knee) can be found. Note that most of these elements are not included in the mechanical models used in this book.

As mentioned before, a number of joints are found within the foot. Two major joint systems located in the rearfoot will be briefly discussed. The *ankle joint* is between the distal ends of tibia and fibula and the talus. The joint is usually considered to act as a simple hinge allowing dorsiflexion and plantarflexion (Inman, 1976). The movement occurs about an axis which passes more or less transversely through the body of the talus (Figure 4.9). The range of motion possible in plantarflexion is about 35° and 25° in dorsiflexion (Lanz & Wachsmuth, 1972). The *subtalar joint* is located between the talus and the calcaneus. The joint allows movement in several anatomical planes about an unstable axis (Figure 4.9). The oblique axis passes from the lateral, inferior part of the calcaneus to the medial side of talus. Motion is primarily that of inversion and eversion of the calcaneus relative to the talus.

The study of these joint motions is a major consideration in running shoe analysis. When filming from the posterior, researchers look at the amount of pronation and supination of a runner's foot during ground contact. *Pronation* usually is referred to as the simultaneous movement

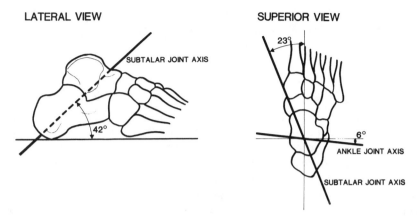

Figure 4.9. The axes of ankle and subtalar joint (Inman, 1976).

of eversion, dorsiflexion, and abduction; *supination* is a combination of inversion, plantarflexion, and adduction. Pronation and supination are, therefore, movements produced by rotations around more than one joint axis.

Ligaments are dense elastic bands which are found in the environment of joints. They connect bone to bone and resist tensile loads. Their stiffness is considerably greater than the stiffness of muscles. Ligaments provide stability to the joints. They guide joint motion and prevent excessive joint movement. Ligaments can be located externally of the joint (e.g., collateral ligaments of the ankle) or inside of a joint (e.g., cruciate ligaments in the knee). The elastic component allows the ligament to come back to its original length after tensile loading. When it is overstretched, however, permanent deformation occurs. The different ligaments in the human body vary considerably in shape and length (see Figure 4.10). The powerful deltoid ligament which supports the medial aspect of the ankle is so strong that even severe tensile stresses produced by excessive eversion will usually not result in a tear of this ligament, but in an avulsion fracture of the medial malleolus. On the other hand, the weaker ligaments at the lateral aspect of the ankle are frequently injured when the ankle is sprained by inversion.

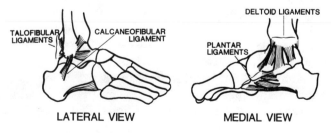

Figure 4.10. The collateral ligaments of the ankle.

Muscle tissue, together with the tendons (connective tissue), makes up individual muscle organs, such as tibialis anterior or gastrocnemius. The main functions of muscle organs are:

- to produce movements (concentric action),
- to decelerate movement (eccentric action), and
- to stabilize the skeletal system (isometric contraction).

Muscles are activated by electric signals and produce movements by exerting forces on their tendons which in turn pull on bones. Most muscles cross at least one joint, and some cross two or more joints. When a muscle contracts, it rotates one articulating bone relative to another. The two bones usually do not move equally in response to the contraction. One is held nearly in place because other muscles contract to pull it in the opposite direction or because its structure makes it less movable. In anatomy, the attachment of a muscle tendon which is closer to the center of the body is called the *origin*. The attachment of the tendon farther away from the center is called the *insertion*.

In producing movements, bones act as levers and joints function as fulcrums of these levers. The muscle forces acting on a lever can generally be divided into propulsive and resistive forces. These forces produce torques, or moments, with respect to a joint. An intended joint movement can only be performed if the sum of the propulsive moments is greater than the sum of the resistive moments. The lever arm and the muscle force are responsible for the moment produced by a muscle and, therefore, for the movement. A muscle attached farther away from a joint will produce a more powerful movement compared to the same muscle attached closer to the fulcrum. If the muscle is inserted closer to the joint, the muscle force has to be bigger to produce the same moment and, therefore, the same movement. Most movements are coordinated by several skeletal muscles acting in groups rather than individually. Consider dorsiflexion of the foot as an example. A muscle that causes a desired action is referred to as an *agonist* or *prime mover*. In this instance, the tibialis anterior muscle (Figure 4.11) is the prime mover. Simultaneously, with the contraction of the agonist, other muscles, called the *antagonists*, are stretched. In this movement, primarily the calf muscles are the antagonists. A particular muscle usually is at various times an agonist or antagonist depending on the movement.

The muscles which act upon the foot can be divided into *extrinsic* and *intrinsic* muscles. The first muscle type has a belly which is located in the leg and has a long tendon which inserts in the foot. In one case (gastrocnemius) the origin is above the knee. The latter type is located entirely in the foot. In this section, only the extrinsic foot muscles will be briefly discussed. These muscles can be grouped according to their functions (Romanes, 1976). It should be noted that most muscles par-

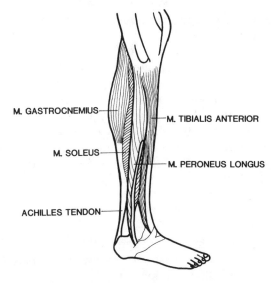

Figure 4.11. Schematic representation of some extrinsic muscles of the foot.

ticipate in different movements. A short summary is presented in the following:

Extensor Group:
The prime movers, located on the lateral anterior side of the tibia and primarily active in dorsiflexion, are the tibialis anterior and the extensor digitorum longus, assisted by the extensor hallucis longus. The latter two muscles are also active in extension of the toes.

Flexor Group:
The important muscles responsible for plantar flexion are the gastrocnemius which originates from the distal, posterior part of the femur and the soleus which lies under the gastrocnemius and originates from the proximal third of tibia and fibula. Their prominent common tendon, the tendo achillis, attaches to the tuber calcanei.

Invertors:
The main invertors of the foot which act in opposition to the peroneal group are the tibialis posterior and tibialis anterior. The tibialis posterior originates from the posterior aspect of tibia and fibula, and its tendon runs behind the medial malleolus. Tibialis anterior, the prominent muscle on the front leg, originates on the lateral side of the tibia and inserts on the plantar surface of the os cuneiform and the first metatarsal. The two muscles are supported by the flexor hallucis longus.

Evertors:
The prime movers for eversion of the foot are the peroneus longus and brevis. They originate from the lateral aspect of the fibula and their tendons run below the lateral malleolus. Peroneus longus attaches to the tuberosity of the first metatarsal and the os cuneiform mediale. Peroneus brevis inserts on the tuberosity of the fifth metataral.

The anatomical structure and anthropometric data within a runner's foot are usually given and cannot be changed. What can be changed, however, is the anatomy of a running shoe. A shoe, or more accurately, certain features of a shoe, can influence lines of action of forces and their lever arms. For instance, a valgus position of a foot or a flatfoot can be corrected by applying orthotics or inserts. The tension in the Achilles tendon during the push-off phase in running can be decreased by a shoe correction. In these cases, the shoe has a positive effect on the loading conditions of the foot. On the other hand, a shoe can have a negative effect on the natural function of the foot during running. Two examples should illustrate this fact in the following:

EXAMPLE 1

The analysis of rearfoot movement shows that when running barefoot, only a minimal amount of initial and maximum pronation is occurring (Nigg & Luethi, 1980). However, most running shoes produce an increase of this pronatory movement. A possible reason for this result is illustrated in Figure 4.12. When running barefoot, the runner's heel touches the ground at about the point where the subtalar joint axis penetrates the

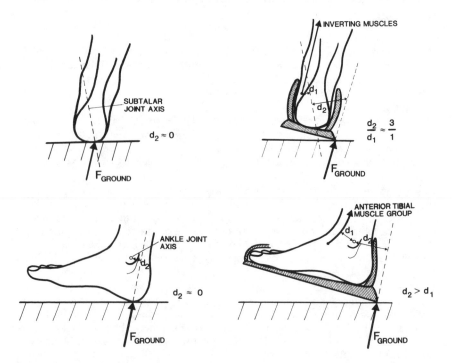

Figure 4.12. The effect of increasing lever arms on the acting moments in ankle and subtalar joints.

calcaneus. This means that the lever-arm of the ground reaction force with respect to the subtalar joint axis is practically zero. Therefore, the ground force does not produce a moment at this joint and hence, initial pronation is small. A shoe with a wide sole flare, as is found in some of today's running shoes, basically increases the lever of the impact forces with respect to the subtalar joint, especially if the outsole is rather stiff. Assuming that the ratio of the lever arms $d_1/d_2 = 3:1$ and the maximum impact force is 1500 N, the inverting muscles should produce a maximum force of about 4500 N in order to equalize the moment produced by the ground reaction force. Because this is not possible, the joint rotates during impact with a high rate of pronation. The inverting muscles and their tendons are stretched with high velocity in the first stage and are supported gradually by the medial ligaments as pronation increases. It is suggested by sport physicians that this medial "slap" of the foot, which occurs at the beginning of every step, could be related to some tibial tendinitis problems.

EXAMPLE 2

A similar example can be shown for the saggital plane (see Figure 4.12). During heel-strike in barefoot running the line of action of the vertical impact force (this component is about 10 to 20 times bigger than the anteroposterior shear force) passes closely to the ankle joint axis. This again means that the moment produced with respect to this axis is small and hence, the forces on the long extensor muscles of the foot are small. Wearing a shoe with a so-called "heel spoiler," however, changes the load situation of these muscles. The effect increases with increasing sole stiffness (Luethi, Nigg, & Bahlsen, 1984). During impact, the moment produced by the ground reaction force and the increased lever arm is too big to be equalized by the anterior tibial muscle group and, therefore, a forefoot slap can occur. This means that these muscles are loaded eccentrically at a high rate, which with time can lead to certain insertion problems at various tendons.

There is no doubt that a running shoe must fulfill special tasks in order to protect the foot and lower extremities. The two examples illustrate how changes in shoe construction can influence internal forces. They underline, as already discussed extensively in chapter 3, that it is not sufficient to study isolated variables. Measurement of external forces with simultaneous analysis of the movement provides information about loading of the internal structure.

5

BENNO M. NIGG
ALEXANDER H. BAHLSEN
JACHEN DENOTH
SIMON M. LUETHI
ALEX STACOFF

Factors influencing kinetic and kinematic variables in running

An ideal analysis of running shoes would determine the relevant variables inside the locomotor system, something not yet done in the past. This analysis is connected with both methodological and logistic problems. The methodological problems are due to the fact that appropriate models, used in applied analysis to estimate internal force and stress, were and are not yet developed. The models currently available are mainly for static or quasistatic movements and are not able to deal with impact forces. The more logistical aspect is connected with the fact that, even if the methodology were available, no study exists showing which of these internal variables would be relevant (e.g., amplitude, loading rate, repetition). One would then have to base the selection of the variables on speculation and intuition. Much of our work is based on an empirical approach with the main emphasis on external variables. We believe that some of these results can provide an improved understanding if the limitation of this approach is appreciated. The variables of interest include the landing impact at the beginning of ground contact, the pronation during the first 50 to 70% of ground contact, and the take-off supination (see Figure 5.1).

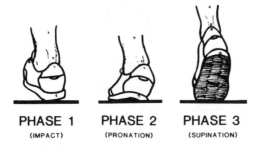

PHASE 1
(IMPACT)

PHASE 2
(PRONATION)

PHASE 3
(SUPINATION)

Figure 5.1. Three phases used in the empirical studies.

Impact Forces

The first measurements, with respect to shoes, in our laboratory were performed in 1972. The measurements were gathered from 5 subjects to whom accelerometers were mounted at the heel, the hip, and the head. The subjects had to run with fixed stride frequency at an average velocity of about 4 m/s, wearing different footwear on different surfaces. The analysis included the measurement of the amplitudes of the accelerations for 10 ground contacts. Figure 5.2 summarizes the mean values for the heel accelerations during heel-toe running. The subjects ran barefoot, had shoes with spikes, or shoes with thin or thick soles. This reflects the time when soft-soled running shoes had just started to appear on the market. The result (about 10 years later) is the starting point for the following comments:

1. The amplitudes of the acceleration at the heel are influenced by footwear on the artificial surface but not on the grass surface.

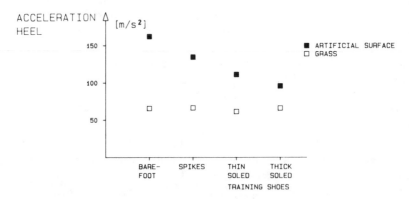

Figure 5.2. Mean values for the heel acceleration in heel-toe running with different footwear on grass and synthetic surface for 5 subjects, 10 trials each at a running velocity of about 4 m/s (Unold, 1974).

2. The acceleration amplitudes are smaller on grass than on the synthetic surface. Even with the softest shoe, the values for the heel acceleration are about 45% higher for the synthetic surface compared to the values on grass.

3. As discussed before, internal forces from these values cannot be determined because additional information would be needed (e.g., knee angle). However, there is some speculation that these acceleration values correspond to impact forces. Furthermore, differences exist for the different shoe and surface conditions. The differences in the accelerations are documented. However, there may be (and most likely are) differences in the kinematic behavior for the different conditions tested.

4. Using impact force values of about 1500 N for heel-toe running with 4 m/s on a hard surface and the average heel acceleration of about 160 m/s² a mass of about 9.4 kg using Newton's $F = m \cdot a$ can be determined. This result corresponds to the values of the effective mass discussed in chapter 3.

These measurements were the beginning of a long development in the understanding of impact forces during heel-toe running. The running shoe in the late 1960s and early 1970s was relatively hard and did not have special elements to cushion the impact forces. This changed drastically in the midseventies, and cushioning was one of the important aspects in the development of new (better) shoes. The left-hand side of Figure 5.3 shows results of impact force measurements for seven different run-

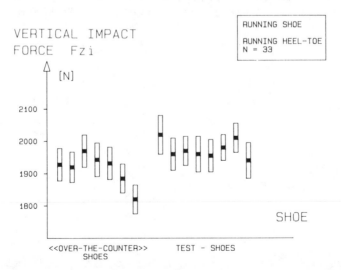

Figure 5.3. Vertical impact force measurements for running shoes. Left: Shoes on the market in 1977 from different companies. Right: Results of a series with especially soft heel cushioning at the same time. Running velocity 4.5 m/s, 33 subjects.

ning shoes from different companies for a running velocity of about 4.5 m/s. On the right-hand side of Figure 5.3, the results are summarized for the same boundary conditions but for a set of test shoes that were developed emphasizing impact force reduction. The graph illustrates that the first series had a range of average vertical impact forces from about 1820 to 1980 N, while the special series had values between 1930 and 2020 N. This result is surprising and is the starting point for further comments.

5. The results of the over-the-counter shoes show a bigger variation than the results of the special test shoes. At that time it was speculated that variation in shoe construction can have an influence on the kinematics of movement during impact which may have an influence on the magnitude of the impact forces. Support for this speculation was received from film analysis for the over-the-counter shoes, showing average values for the initial pronation of the rearfoot angle ranging from 6 to 9°. It was assumed that these differences have an effect on the internal impact forces.

6. One would have expected that the special cushioning series would reduce the vertical impact force peaks compared to the over-the-counter shoes. Because this is not the case, one has to try to understand the reason for this result. A possible explanation is illustrated in Figure 5.4.

This figure represents the results of a test series which compares maximal impact forces in running heel-toe with a running velocity of about 3.5 m/s for 13 test subjects (26 trials, left and right) with results of maximum impact forces of a drop test (m = 5 kg, v = 2 m/s) performed with

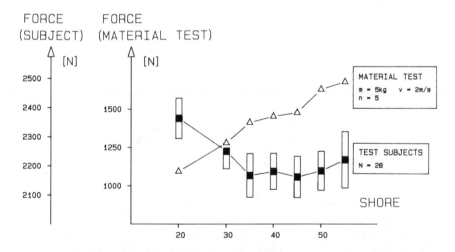

Figure 5.4. Results of an impact test (first impact) and a test with subjects running heel-toe with a set of identical shoes where the hardness of the shoe sole was systematically varied between 20 and 55 shore.

the same set of shoes. The shoes were identical in their construction but varied systematically in the hardness of the midsole at the rear part of the foot with shore values of 20, 30, 35, 40, 45, 50, and 55. The material tests were performed with the MODYME for the different shoes. The general results of these two experiments with the same set of shoes are different. The results of the material test suggest that the shoe with the lowest force, shoe with shore 20, is the softest. However, the results of the test with test subjects suggest that the softest shoe would be a shoe with a sole hardness of 35-45 shore. This result is, again, the trigger for several reflections:

7. Impact forces of the running test series increase for materials with shore 30 and even more with shore 20. This can be explained by a "bottoming out" effect. The material is too soft and is totally compressed relatively fast, which then results in high force amplitudes.

8. A determination of internal impact forces would provide more relevant (and maybe slightly changed) results. However, the basic finding of an optimal sole hardness would not change.

9. The *optimal range* depends on various aspects. It is very much an individual range depending on running velocity and running style which includes the knee angle and the touch down velocity as the most important variables. Subjects running with hard landing obviously need a harder shoe than subjects with a very soft landing. Because the curve for the subject test in Figure 5.4 rises quickly for softer shoes (left side) but very slowly for increasing hardness (right side), it seems reasonable to shift the optimal range slightly to the harder side. Having a shoe with a slightly higher shore value obviously does less harm than having a shoe with a too soft sole. In this example, it would mean that a change from shore 35 to 25 would increase the external vertical impact forces from 2170 N to about 2300 N. However, changing from 35 to 45 shore would in this example not affect the vertical impact forces. Even a change to shore 55 has only a small effect on the vertical impact peak.

10. The reflections and calculations in chapter 3 suggest that measurements of external impact forces are correlated with the corresponding internal impact forces if the lever-arm of the external force, with respect to the joint, is not too large. It can, therefore, be assumed that the external impact forces are a good indicator for the relevant load at the joint. If this assumption is correct, one can conclude that the material test used in this example is not at all relevant with respect to impact force reduction in running. It shows nothing else than what one already knows from shore measurement and does not describe the bottoming out effect seen in the tests with test subjects.

Furthermore, it can be concluded that every test which uses smaller masses and/or smaller velocities will measure the same results and will, therefore, not quantify relevant information with respect to running shoe cushioning. This example shows that results from material tests should be used appropriately, namely, to quantify information with respect to material. If one wants to use them for a simulation of internal impact forces, much more information must be included. No such test exists today. Impact tests as used in various places should, therefore, not be used to assess the quality of a running shoe. Furthermore, it can be stated that softness in the heel sole of a running shoe is not identical with hardness or softness expressed by the shore value or experienced by pressing the fingers in the heel material. It is an optimization problem.

Hardness of material is just one of several factors that influence impact peaks in running shoes. Another factor is a change in the geometry of the shoe sole. One strategy runners can use to adapt to changed external conditions may be, as mentioned earlier, a change in the positioning of the foot and leg at impact. Figure 5.5 illustrates such a strategy for dif-

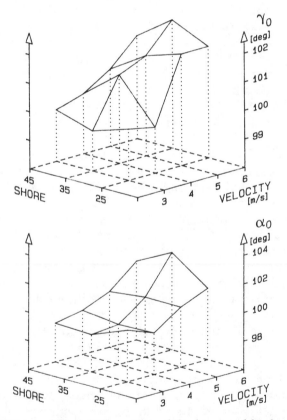

Figure 5.5. Change of the initial position of the leg α and heel γ for different velocities and shore values of the shoes for 16 subjects running at different velocities (posterior view).

ferent running velocities and hardnesses of the shoe sole. The result shows that the leg and foot are more everted with increasing running velocity. However, there is no systematic change for the hardnesses used. The external forces increase with increasing velocity. The subjects in this experiment changed the position of the foot to a more everted position for increasing load. The initial area of contact is, therefore, decreasing in this example with increasing load.

In order to understand this result, one has to understand the connection between contact area and the hardness of an element. The spring constant describing the hardness of an element is proportional to the area of contact. An increasing area of contact increases the spring constant and, therefore, the hardness of the element. If the subjects increase their rearfoot angle, they decrease the area of contact. Doing so, they make the contacting element softer. It could be that this experimental result is an involuntary adaptation to the higher loading forces. On the other hand, one must use softer materials for increased areas of contact between surface and shoe at impact.

Further important factors which may have an influence on external impact forces are the running velocity and the mass distribution. Their influence on the impact peaks are discussed in the following two experiments:

Experiment 1. Sixteen test subjects were analyzed for the influence of running velocity and sole hardness. The subjects ran (heel-toe) with the velocities 3, 4, 5, and 6 m/s ($\pm$ 0.2 m/s) over a force platform using three identical shoes where only the hardness of the midsole was varied (25, 35, and 45 shore). Note that the second factor (hardness) was already studied in the experiment discussed in Figure 5.4. The results of this study for the vertical impact peak and the maximal loading rate are represented in Figure 5.6.

Experiment 2. Twenty-one test subjects were analyzed to measure the influence of masses added to the foot, the lower leg, and the hip. The subjects were running (heel-toe) with a velocity of 4 m/s ($\pm$ 0.4 m/s). The additional masses at the foot were added at the outside of the heel, at the distal end of the tibia for the leg, and in a backpack for the hip. The results for the vertical and horizontal impact peaks are illustrated in Figure 5.7. The results for these two experiments may help to explain external impact peaks better and are again the starting point for several comments.

11. The averages for the impact peaks for the experiment with the additional masses did not differ from a statistical point of view. However, it is worth discussing the various cases one after the other. The maximal additional mass of 0.1 kg at the *foot* is assumed to be about 1.5% of the effective mass. One can, therefore, not expect more than an increase of about 1.5% of the impact peak of 1430 N with no mass, which would correspond to an increase of about 22 N. The value

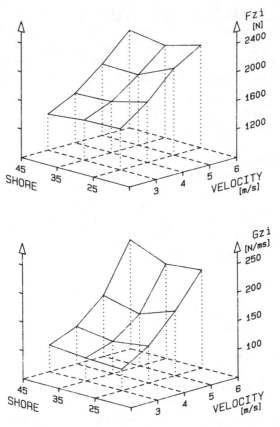

Figure 5.6. Vertical impact peaks F_{zi} and maximal loading rate G_{zi} as a function of running velocity and hardness of the midsole (16 subjects).

measured was 1463 N which is slightly higher than the theoretical value. However, both changes move in the same direction. The additional maximal mass at the *tibia* is 0.6 kg which corresponds to about 9% of the effective mass. One would theoretically expect an increase of about 130 N for the vertical impact peak. However, the impact peak in the experiment decreases slightly from 1430 N to 1417 N. Therefore, the subjects must have used another strategy in order to reduce these impact forces. The film analysis showed that the vertical touch down velocities were reduced from 0.99 m/s to 0.92 m/s which corresponds to a change of about 7%. The fact that for the additional masses the impact peak did not change can be explained by the change in the impact velocity. The additional mass at the hip can be assumed to add about 25% to the effective mass which would correspond to an increase of about 360 N. The experimental increase is only 53 N. The velocity did not change. However, the knee angle changed (about

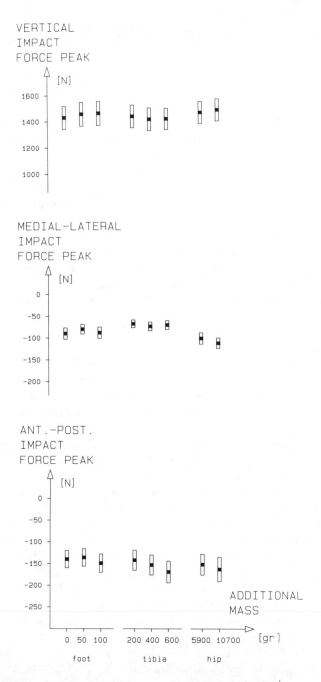

Figure 5.7. Vertical and horizontal impact peaks for running at 4 m/s (± 0.4 m/s) with and without additional masses at the foot, the leg, and the hip (21 subjects).

4 degrees). This corresponds to a change in the effective mass of about 1 to 1.5 kg which can explain most of the missing increase. Note that these comments are made for the mean values for 21 subjects. An individual analysis shows that this strategy is subject dependent. However, the majority solved the problem in this way.

12. The variation of the hardness of the sole (for this shoe construction), between 25 and 45 shore, showed little influence on the impact force peaks. This result is in line with the result illustrated in Figure 5.6. The fact that the optimal plateau has shifted a little towards smaller shore values may be connected with the thicker shoe sole of the test shoes in this experiment.

13. The running velocity has a dominant influence on the impact force peaks. They are between 1300 and 1400 N for 3 m/s and between 2090 and 2240 N for 6 m/s of running velocity. This result makes it evident that cushioning is recommended for high velocities of running or jogging. It also suggests that cushioning for lower velocities or, better, for lower forces, may be less critical.

14. The previous comments can also be made for the maximal loading rate. The only difference lies in the fact that the relation between impact force peak F_{zi} and maximal loading rate G_{zi} is not linear as discussed in chapter 2.

15. Shore and additional mass variation did not have an outstanding influence on the impact force peaks. Theoretically, these variations should have an influence as explained earlier. The fact that they do not have one could be explained by assuming that each athlete has a certain level of tolerance for impact forces which he or she allows. The strategies selected to fulfill these requirements may then be different, but they certainly must have an effect which can be seen in the kinematic analysis (Nigg & Denoth, 1980; Clarke et al., 1983). One may speculate that the whole procedure of adaptation looks like an automatic protection mechanism (Nigg et al., 1974).

16. The results in Figures 5.6 and 5.7 with respect to hardness and impact force peaks do not agree with the results from Frederick and co-workers (1984). The results of their study were that thickness (heel height) and hardness have an influence on impact force peaks, but flare does not have one. The influence of thickness was not studied in the two experiments. However, results of the Biomechanics Laboratory in Zurich (Denoth et al., 1984) for midsole thicknesses between 0 and 25 mm and shore values of 30, 45, and 60 (measurements with 20 subjects) did not show the expected difference of impact force peaks for different midsole thicknesses. Furthermore, the results of our experiments (see Figure 5.6) did not show an influence of the hardness (shore values) in the analyzed range which is iden-

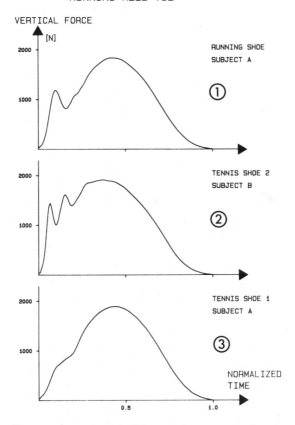

Figure 5.8. Different types of vertical impact force curves for running depending on the subject-shoe combination.

tical to Frederick's range. Based on the theoretical considerations in chapter 3, we expect that flare should have an effect even though we did not measure this influence. The fundamental difference in these results may be explained by the fact that Frederick's results are based on impact tests with an impact tester, while our results are based on tests with test subjects. If this assumption is correct, this would again underline that material tests have to be used with extreme caution and that the athlete reacts on various constructions of running shoes with his or her own movement strategies which probably operate using some kind of stress level. This level is expected to be movement velocity and/or shoe geometry dependent for the ranges studied in these experiments.

Using the explanations and comments with respect to impact, one can develop a clear summary of the important factors. The most important conclusion is that an athlete has various possibilities to influence these impact forces, and that they are widely used. Another important finding is that changes in geometry have a much bigger influence than changes in material (shore). The reported results and reflections seem to be an important step forward in respect to the understanding of impact forces in heel-toe running. However, some limiting comments have to be added to complete the picture. Impact peaks are not always visible (Cavanagh & Lafortune, 1980; Luethi, 1983). This is one reason for using the maximal loading rate for impact analysis. However, the aspect which is much more interesting is the reason for the occurrence or absence of such clear peaks.

Furthermore, some athlete-shoe combinations have double peaks as illustrated in Figure 5.8 for running. Luethi (1983) subdivided the most frequent types of curves into Type 1 with one impact peak, Type 2 with a double impact peak, and Type 3 with no impact peak visible. More categories may be possible. However, he states that with this subdivision most of the vertical force curves can be classified for heel-toe running. Cavanagh and Lafortune (1980) assign the Type 3 curves to midfoot landing and the Type 1 curves to heel landing. A careful analysis of our experimental results showed Type 3 curves for clear heel landing as well as for flat landing. This is still not clearly understood. At this time we can speculate (Nigg, 1983) the following as explanations:

1. The first dominant peak in Type 1 and 2 curves may be caused by a heel strike.
2. The occurrence of two impact peaks in the Type 2 curves may be caused by an impact-type landing of the forefoot or a lateral slapping of the midfoot and/or forefoot.
3. The absence of an impact peak in the Type 3 curves may be caused by a midfoot landing as suggested by Cavanagh and Lafortune (1980), or may be produced by the stiffness of the sole.

Explanations 1 and 2 are easy to accept. However, explanation 3 is not really an explanation but more of a description of a boundary effect. This point is clearly not well understood and needs more research. The fact that stiffer shoes (e.g., tennis shoes) which are not designed for jogging or running produce Type 2 and 3 curves illustrates another problem of impact force analysis. Based on the criteria commonly used for experimental impact force analysis and cushioning, one would describe a Type 3 curve as an ideal one. However, in reality, one would not use tennis shoes for running. This result underlines the importance of developing a model which allows the quantification of internal impact forces using geometrical information combined with ground reaction force.

Pronation

Pronation or overpronation is speculated as being one reason for runners' injuries as stated in chapters 1 and 2. It is, therefore, logical to study the movement of the shoe (rearfoot angle) and the movement in the ankle joint (Achilles tendon angle). In the example (see Figure 5.9) the subject lands in a position with a rearfoot angle of about 90° and an Achilles tendon angle of about 186°. The subject, therefore, lands in a slightly pronated position. The rearfoot position or the angle of maximum pronation is about 71° and the maximum Achilles tendon angle is about 212°. The maximal change in the Achilles tendon angle which can be used to describe this pronatory movement is about 26°. There is no doubt that this extreme overpronation has to be reduced. The question is, How can the shoe influence pronation? There are, of course, several ways to control pronation by varying the shoe construction. One of the most commonly used strategies is the use of a medial support. The questions to be answered are: *If* a medial arch support can influence pronation during heel-toe running and *how* can this be done. For this purpose, a series of five identical running shoes were used. The only variable which was systematically varied was the medial support. Shoe 1 was a shoe with no support at all. Shoes 2 to 5 were shoes where a medial support was systematically positioned from anterior (Shoe 2) to posterior (Shoe 5) as illustrated in Figure 5.10.

The material of the medial support was an elastic cork. The experiments were performed with 20 subjects and a running speed of about 4 m/s. The variables analyzed and discussed in this context are the initial changes of the rearfoot $\Delta\gamma_{10}$, the Achilles tendon angle $\Delta\beta_{10}$, and the total pronation $\Delta\beta_{pro}$. The results for barefoot and for the five shoe conditions are summarized and shown in Figure 5.10.

The result shows that a medial support influences the initial pronation of the rearfoot and the Achilles tendon angle. The initial pronation (about 30 ms) in the rearfoot angle, $\Delta\gamma_{10}$, changes from 6.9° for no support to

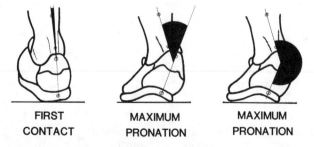

| FIRST | MAXIMUM | MAXIMUM |
| CONTACT | PRONATION | PRONATION |

Figure 5.9. Illustration of pronation for a heavy pronator, using two conventional angles.

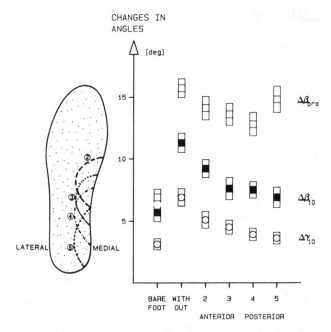

Figure 5.10. The results for pronation for barefoot and shoes with systematically varied location of medial support for 20 subjects running heel-toe with 4 m/s. Shore value for midsole was between 35 and 40.

3.6° for the most posterior position. The initial change of the Achilles tendon angle is 11.3° for shoes without medial support and 6.9° for the shoe with support at the most posterior position. Both results for the most posterior position are in the same order of magnitude as the values for barefoot running for this group. The differences due to varied positioning of the medial support in the total pronation are rather small (15.7° for the unsupported shoe and 12.8° for the position 4) and not even a similar trend, as for the initial values, can be seen. Additionally, there is for all shoes a big difference compared to barefoot. These results are reason for several comments.

1. Obviously, a medial support reduces the initial pronation if placed in the posterior part of the midfoot. Medial supports which are placed too much toward the forefoot have much less effect in reducing initial pronation. The location of medial supports in today's running shoes is, in many cases, too much toward the forefoot. Medial support placed correctly reduces the initial pronation and, therefore, the initial loading rate of the structures controlling pronation. This effect is certainly welcome and is expected to reduce pain and injuries.

2. The result that the medial support clearly did not reduce total pronation is surprising and was not expected at all. We expected that there

would be a clear difference between shoes without and shoes with medial support with respect to total pronation.

3. The two results, a clear effect on initial and a rather small effect on total pronation, needs an explanation. The small effect on total pronation could be explained when studying the midsole. The relatively stiff support sits on a relatively soft foundation, a midsole with a hardness of about 30 to 40 shore. For such a construction, the location of this support is of minor importance because the stiffer support will sink into the softer midsole material under the high forces during stance. Therefore, a significant effect will not result. A mechanical explanation for the initial pronation could be that the support material reacts harder on impact forces, because of viscoelastic factors, in comparison to the active phase. A second explanation could be that the geometry is changed. However, this explanation is not completely satisfactory and it may well be that a medial support at the more posterior part of the shoe produces a psychological barrier. The athlete feels the support and moves more carefully.

4. *However*, knowing the results of this experiment one has to be careful in using medial supports in order to influence pronation. The results show that (a) medial supports can influence initial pronation significantly, and (b) medial supports may have only little influence on total pronation. The results do not suggest that medial supports are worthless, but rather suggest that their value is in the reduction of the loading rate and not in the reduction of the maximum pronation. Furthermore, it may well be that other aspects, such as comfort, are also important with respect to medial support. Because medial support may not reveal all the effects one expected from them with respect to pronation, other possible strategies have to be analyzed and discussed.

Another method of influencing pronation is the use of different material hardness for the midsole. In order to study this effect, an experiment was performed using three shoes which were identical except for the hardness of the midsole (25, 35, and 45 shore). Sixteen subjects ran heel-toe with different running velocities (3, 4, 5, and 6 m/s $\pm$ 0.2 m/s). They were filmed from posterior as described in chapter 2. The results for the initial and total pronation are summarized in Figure 5.11. The initial pronation includes by definition the contact time. A variable which does not include the contact time but describes the average initial loading rate is the average initial angular velocity, $\dot{\beta}_{10}$. For experiments with varying running velocity, this variable will be used. The average initial angular velocity for the Achilles tendon angle shows increasing values for increasing velocity as well as for increasing hardness of the midsole. The total pronation $\Delta\beta_{pro}$ shows a different general result for the influence of the midsole hardness, but the same general shape for increasing velocities. The change

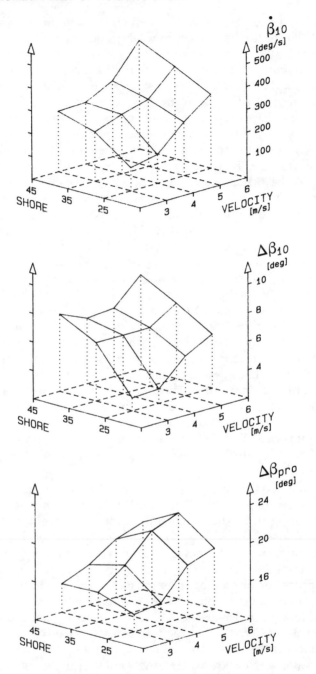

Figure 5.11. Influence of running velocity and midsole hardness on initial pronation, initial angular velocity, and total pronation for the Achilles tendon angle ($n = 16$).

from 25 to 35 shore shows an increase in total pronation for all running velocities. The change from 35 to 45 shore shows no effect for small velocities but a decrease of total pronation for higher velocities. Once again, this result for total pronation was not expected and the whole experiment asks for additional comments.

5. The generally increasing initial angular velocity and total pronation is connected with the higher forces acting for faster running velocities. Note that this result is not in agreement with results published by Bates and co-workers (1978).

6. The increasing initial angular velocity as a result of harder midsole can be explained by a stiffer lever arm system. A softer shoe sole would first compress and then rotate; a harder shoe sole would compress less and rotate faster. Therefore, soft heel material, especially in the region of first contact which is usually the lateral side of the rear part of the shoe, reduces the initial pronation.

7. The result for the total pronation can be explained as follows: Changing from 25 to 35 increases the maximum pronation because of the increased angular velocity (pronation velocity). The midsole material is not hard enough to resist the pronation movement which results in a high maximum pronation. However, if the midsole becomes harder (shore 45), it can resist the pronatory movement better which results in a smaller maximum pronation.

8. This result leads to the conclusion that (a) the material which should absorb the shock should be softer than the rest of the midsole material and located where the impact occurs, and (b) the material of the midsole should be harder to reduce pronation.

There is no doubt that the hardness of the impact absorbing part has to be adjusted to aspects such as area of contact, style of running, and velocity of running. These comments are supported by the observation that our measurements with subjects wearing running shoes from different companies in the last 5 years show that the initial pronation is slightly reduced while the total pronation is clearly increased. The results suggest a construction of a shoe as illustrated in Figure 5.12. The subjects land on the lateral part of the rearfoot.

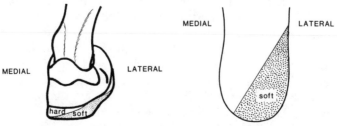

Figure 5.12. Possible solution of shoe which addresses the requirements of reduction of pronation using a double density sole in the rear part as well as a slightly rounded lateral heel.

The material which is soft compresses. The line of action of the ground reaction force moves toward the subtalar joint which reduces the lever-arm and, therefore, the moment. The foot pronates more slowly. In contrast, the resistance against pronation increases because of the harder material, and the pronation can be reduced. Experimental data with results of 2 test subjects running in their shoes and with a prototype shoe constructed in this way are illustrated in Figure 5.13. The results show that in both cases, the runners are heavy pronators, and that with this special shoe the pronation could be drastically reduced.

9. The considerations in this chapter lead to an additional speculation: The current strategy to use a midsole material which is relatively soft and to reinforce the sole with harder elements in locations where certain effects should occur, is only one, and possibly not the optimal solution of sole construction. It is speculated that a solution with a harder midsole and softer cushioning material used in the appropriate locations would solve cushioning and pronation problems more adequately. The side effect, that flexibility may decrease, can be overcome by special geometrical solutions of the forefoot.

10. The results with respect to the influence of midsole hardness on total pronation do not agree with the results published by Clarke and co-workers (1984). They state that "shoes having midsoles softer than 35 durometer will allow significantly more maximum pronation and total rearfoot movement." There are, of course, various ways to explain these differences. The one we favor most is that the overall hardness and geometry of the sole is not only determined by the hardness of the midsole but by the geometrical construction of the total sole. We speculate that the soles of our shoes, overall, were somewhat harder. This would mean that the shoes from Clarke with shore 35 correspond to our shoes with shore 25. If this is correct, then the contradiction does not exist. This, again, underlines the importance of the geometrical solution of a shoe.

There are many different ways to control pronation, fulfilling at the same time the requirements of impact reduction. Clarke and co-workers (1984) analyzed the influence of heel flare in connection with midsole hardness. They found that shoes having less flare allow more total pronation. However, Cavanagh (1980) and Subotnick (1981) expressed the opinion that increased medial flare can reduce pronation, while lateral flare is not beneficial because of the increased lever arm. The two statements are obviously contradictory. Based on our theoretical and experimental results, we conclude that lateral flare does increase pronation. Obviously, this question needs more research.

A systematic analysis of factors influencing pronation in running was presented by Stacoff and Kaelin (1983), including shoe mechanical factors such as sole thickness and stiffness, geometry, heel counter, and or-

SUBJECT A   SUBJECT B

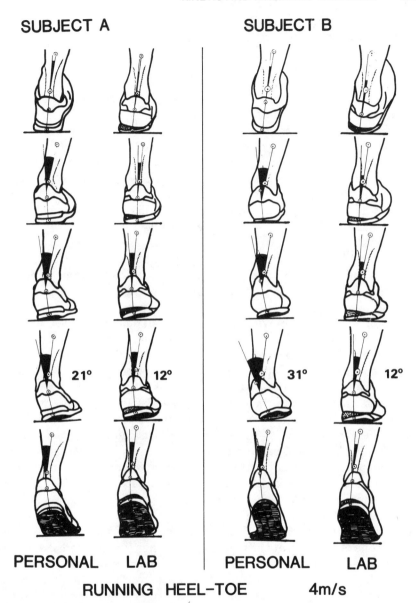

21°   12°   31°   12°

PERSONAL   LAB   PERSONAL   LAB

RUNNING HEEL–TOE   4m/s

Figure 5.13. The effect of a shoe with a double density sole and a slightly rounded heel for two runners which had excessive pronation in their commonly used shoes.

thotics; biomechanical factors such as surface, touch down velocity, and foot position; and biomedical factors, such as foot type and laxity of ligaments. It illustrates the complexity of the problem and the variety of possible solutions.

Take-Off Supination

Take-off supination, which means a rolling over on the outside of the forefoot during take-off combined with a medial rotation of the rearfoot, is speculated as being one possible reason for Achilles tendon pain. Furthermore, take-off supination may have a negative effect on performance because force is applied in a direction which does not contribute to the forward movement. It is, therefore, meaningful to study the factors influencing take-off supination and some strategies for avoiding it.

The take-off angle for subjects running barefoot is relatively close to 180°. However, take-off angles for running with running shoes were measured in the range between 160 and 180° and quite frequently around 170°. Therefore, the shoe is mainly responsible for this take-off supination. Results for different running velocities and shore values did not show significant differences. The mean values were all between 166.6 and 169.1° which is the same order of magnitude. Both variables, running velocity and hardness of the midsole, appear not to be relevant with respect to take-off supination.

In another experiment with 44 cases, with no pain or injuries, we analyzed the influence of an additional medial support in a conventional running shoe. In this project we found that an additional medial support increased the take-off supination an average of about 5° (172.2 ± 7.4° for normal running shoes and 167.1 ± 9.5° for the same shoes with an additional medial support). A similar result for the take-off angle was found in a project where the medial support was placed in different locations. The results for this experiment are illustrated in Figure 5.14. Obviously, there seems to be a trend toward increasing the take-off supination when the medial support is located more toward the rearfoot. It is assumed that the subject lands on the lateral part of the sole and rolls over to the medial side. A medial support may produce a reaction leading the movement to the outside of the forefoot which results in a take-off supination (Segesser & Nigg, 1980). The logical consequence of these considerations is an experiment where the findings for the medial support are included, and a mechanical help to reduce the forefoot supination is added. This experiment was conducted with four identical shoes (Shoe 4 of Figure 5.10) with a lateral support varying from the posterior to the anterior part of the shoe. Twelve test subjects performed heel-toe running at a speed of about 4 m/s. The results of this experiment (see Figure 5.15) show that geometrical alterations of the forefoot of the shoe can have a significant influence on the take-off angle. Obviously, the best result for this series was a shoe with the lateral support in the forefoot, while the lateral support in the rearfoot did not produce a change compared to no lateral support (see Figure 5.15). A lateral support is, of course, not

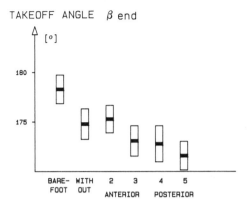

Figure 5.14. Influence of medial support on the take-off angle in running (20 subjects running heel-toe with 4 m/s).

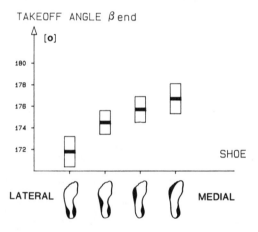

Figure 5.15. Influence of a lateral support on the take-off supination during running heel-toe (12 subjects, 24 trials, 4 m/s).

the only strategy to use. However, the results from the experiments suggest that geometrical solutions would be more effective in reducing take-off supination. One additional geometrical strategy is the use of leading grooves in the (not too soft) midsole material of the forefoot.

Other strategies can be applied to influence take-off supination. The same can be said about control of pronation and impact reduction. The examples discussed show the effect of some changes in running shoe construction and may help to increase the general understanding. Further research is needed to study the effect of other construction strategies.

6

BENNO M. NIGG

Some comments for runners

Lectures on the topic "Biomechanical Aspects of Running Shoes" are quite popular these days. Personally, I like giving these lectures because we have an important obligation to provide everyone who is interested with the knowledge of our research in running shoes. Usually such a lecture is followed by a discussion, and in most cases, one of the first questions asked is, "What is the best running shoe today?" This question is legitimate, but this one question is not enough. After reading, studying, and understanding the contents of the first five chapters of this book, the following *two* basic questions arise:

1. How can I find out which shoe I should buy for my specific running requirements?
2. How can I prevent running injuries without quitting my beloved sport?

In the following pages I have attempted to answer these two questions in a simple and practical way much like a recipe. Therefore, this part of the book is different from the first five chapters where the scientific research approach, based on analytical thinking, experimental results, and systematic analysis, was used. In this chapter, these findings are applied to everyday situations in the world of competition, of injuries, and of miles and kilometers. In doing so, we allow more speculation enabling us to apply the knowledge to the runners' needs.

Which Shoe Should I Buy?

The answer to this question is found in the previous chapters in which the main functions of a shoe were discussed. A good running shoe should

- reduce impact forces
- control pronation, and
- control take-off supination.

Of course, there are other considerations such as color, fashion, flexibility, and price. However, biomechanically, with respect to load on the runner's body and subsequent injuries, the former three functions are of utmost importance.

IMPACT FORCES

The results of our studies showed that there are different groups of runners: the "heavy pounders" who land with high impact forces; the "soft" runners who run with small impact forces (like cats); and, of course, those in between. For soft runners, impact reduction is not relevant at all because the problem of impact forces is solved in using an appropriate running style. However, for a heavy pounder, protection is very important. The question then arises as to how a runner can find out to which group he or she belongs. One method is to *listen*! Heavy pounders can hear the heel contact. I suggest to every runner that he or she go to a marathon once, not as a participant but as a spectator, and listen to the athletes. The noise (impact noise) of quite a few athletes is impressive. Another way to quantify the effect of impact forces is to be aware of the effect of each impact. If the runner can feel the shock in the lower extremities and even in the low back, he or she probably belongs to the heavy pounder group.

Because the soft runners do not need special cushioning or reduction of the impact forces, we will concentrate on the heavy pounders and those who feel that cushioning is important for them. How can they find out which shoe should buy and whether a shoe does the job of cushioning appropriately? This is relatively difficult. I can easily explain what *not* to do: Do not take a shoe and press your fingers in the material and think that the shoe cushions more if your fingers penetrate more. Do not stand on the heel of the shoe pressing with the foot on the shoe and think that if the shoe feels softer, it cushions better than if it feels harder. Both "tests" do not tell anything with respect to cushioning. The only reliable test would be to stamp with the heel onto the ground. If that hurts, the shoe may be too soft. We know from our results that one of the critical points in the impact cushioning is the bottoming out effect. Furthermore, we know that cushioning is an optimization procedure. Too soft as well as too hard heel materials can have negative effects. However, the impact forces increase faster on the soft side of the optimum and slower on the hard one which means that it is *safer to take a harder shoe* than a softer one. Thus, heavy pounder runners are better protected if they select a relatively hard-heeled running shoe.

PRONATION

The results of several thousand foot contacts analyzed over the last 12 years showed that a runner pronates more running with running shoes than running barefoot, and that overpronation frequently occurs. Again, go to a marathon and watch your fellow runners from the rear. What you can see with respect to pronation and overpronation is shocking. Some runners give the impression that they are standing beside their shoes! Athletes with pronation values of more than 30° are not unusual.

These suggestions will help you proceed in checking the aspect of pronation when buying a new running shoe. Take a friend with you who knows your running style. Wear the shoe, and let your friend control your pronation. He or she can easily see if there is overpronation. Note, however, if one shoe of one company produces an overpronation this does not mean that all other shoes of the same company do the same. If a shoe shows overpronation, put this shoe aside and try another. Generally, shoes that are soft (too soft) in the midfoot area allow more pronation or overpronation. A runner with an overpronation problem should, therefore, look for a shoe that has little or even negative flare on the outside of the heel. A rounded heel, for instance, usually reduces pronation. Furthermore, that runner should avoid shoes that are soft in the medial part of the midsole. A medial arch support on a somewhat harder midsole may reduce pronation. There are two aspects to control: Attempt to reduce the moments producing the pronation that can be done on the outside of the heel; and stop the pronatory movement which can be done at the inside.

SUPINATION

Take-off supination means a rolling over the outside of the forefoot during take-off. Most runners do not do that running barefoot. However, many of the shoes produce some take-off supination which may be 20 to 25°. This take-off supination can be detected by observing the athlete from the rear. Note that it is easier to first check pronation and then take-off supination rather than trying to observe both at the same time. The new developments in running shoe construction deal mainly with the first two aspects: impact reduction and control of pronation. (Take-off supination was somewhat neglected.) Excessive take-off supination can be reduced with a lateral support in the forefoot. Some shoes do have such a support. If not, it can easily be added. There are other strategies in shoe construction, for instance, groove treads in the midsole, which are not obvious for a runner. The practical advice for the runner is therefore rather sparse.

ADDITIONAL COMMENTS

- These recommendations are made for heel-toe runners who make up the majority of the runners' population.
- An attentive reader may have realized that we feel that a too soft running shoe may do more harm than a too hard one. The approach in the last decade to use a soft midsole and to add more stable or harder parts to produce a special effect or support is not the ideal approach. I would recommend just the opposite and use a harder midsole and insert the softer elements where needed (e.g., lateral heel).
- Reduction of internal impact forces is usually compensated for with an increase in pronation and a reduction of pronation by an increase of impact forces. This is not a necessity but rather a reality. Theoretically, a round heel (outside) with a thick and soft padding would reduce both internal impact forces and pronation. However, most shoes are not constructed in this way. Therefore, in each situation a careful analysis is necessary to decide which of these factors are important and thus to avoid new problems.
- A similar comment can describe the connection between pronation and take-off supination. A decrease in pronation is usually followed by an increase in take-off supination. Special constructions or inserts are needed in order to control this.
- A runner's clinic, providing on-line information about the problems discussed in this chapter and about internal forces would be extremely helpful in selecting appropriate running footwear, especially for problem-ridden athletes.

Prevention of Running Injuries

The comments regarding the prevention of running injuries are similar to the comments on the selection of shoes. One has to carefully check impact, pronation, and take-off supination. The shoe itself is obviously one means of influencing these three aspects. However, there are other means of preventing injuries. The impact forces can be influenced by the running style (soft landing) and the surface. Running on grass reduces the impact force more than a running shoe is able to do on asphalt. Another aspect which is frequently neglected is the active contribution of the musculoskeletal system in the control of pronation. Every runner should keep in mind that special exercises for his or her lower extremities, and especially for the ankle joint, may be one strategy to use to reduce injuries.

In summary, an athlete can use external elements to influence load and stress on his body. The two most important ones are the running shoe and the surface. On the other hand, he or she can use internal elements which are muscles, tendons, ligaments, and so forth, and his or her running style. Careful exercise and control of these elements is an important factor in the attempt to reduce running injuries.

Sport physicians attribute many running injuries to one of the three mentioned aspects: impact forces, overpronation, and oversupination. Most of them are acute injuries. A large percentage of these acute injuries are connected with overpronation and oversupination. Fewer are assumed to be connected with impact forces. However, we speculate that too high impact forces may be responsible for long-term effects which may result in chronic injuries, for instance, damage of cartilage in a joint. Acute injuries are, therefore, only one aspect of importance. Chronic injuries may be more critical in a long-term perspective.

Another injury-prevention consideration is the mileage. The human body is not primarily constructed to run and jog. It is certainly not built to frequently run long distances on asphalt. However, for so many runners this activity is a much needed compensation to the psychological stress and to the physiological passivity in the working environment. Consequently, the solution is an optimization. It may well be that the mechanical stress level can be kept in a lower range by adapting and/or reducing the mileage. The shoe can certainly take over part, but only part, of stress reduction.

References

ARCAN, N., Brull, M., & Simkin, A. (1976). Mechanical parameters, describing the standing posture, based on the foot-ground pressure pattern. In P.V. Komi (Ed.), *Biomechanics V-B* (pp. 415-425). Baltimore: University Park Press.

ARITOMI, H., Morita, M., & Yonemoto, K. (1983). A simple method of measuring the footsole pressure of normal subjects using pre-scale pressure-detecting sheets. *Journal of Biomechanics*, **16**, 157-165.

BATES, B.T., Osternig, L.R., & Mason, B. (1978). Lower extremity function during the support phase of running. In E. Asmussen & K. Jorgensen (Eds.), *Biomechanics VI-A* (pp. 31-39). Baltimore: University Park Press.

BATES, B.J., Osternig, L.R., Mason, B.R., & James, S.L. (1979). Functional variability of the lower extremity during the support phase of running. *Medicine and Science in Sports*, **11**, 328-331.

BAUMANN, J.N., & Procter, P. (1985). Camera speeds in gait analysis. In D. Winter (Ed.), *Biomechanics IX-A* (pp. 280-286). Champaign, IL: Human Kinetics Publishers.

BAUMANN, W., & Stucke, H. (1980). Sportspezifische belastungen aus der sicht der biomechanik [Sport specific load from a biomechanical point of view]. In H. Cotta, H. Krahl, & K. Steinbrueck (Eds.), *Die Belastungstoleranz des Bewegungsapparates* (pp. 55-64). Stuttgart: Thieme.

BIERREGAARD, S.A. (1945). Semelle interieure orthopedique. [Orthopaedic inserts]. *Brevet d'invention*, Nr. 913.372. Paris: Ministere de la production industrielle.

BOLLIGER, A. (1979). Seid nett zu euren gelenken [Be polite to your joints]. *Smash Tennis Magazine*, **1**, 41-43.

BONSTINGEL, R.W., Morehouse, C.A., & Niebel, B.W. (1975). Torques developed by different types of shoes on various playing surfaces. *Medicine and Science in Sports*, **7**, 127-131.

BOWERS, K.D., & Martin, R.B. (1974). Impact absorption, new and old Astroturf at West Virginia University. *Medicine and Science in Sports*, **6**, 217-221.

BOWERS, K.D., & Martin, R.B. (1975). Cleat surface friction on new and old Astroturf. *Medicine and Science in Sport*, **7**, 132.

BRAMWELL, S.T., Requa, R.K., & Garrick, J.C. (1972). High school football injuries: A pilot comparison of playing surfaces. *Medicine and Science in Sports*, **4**, 166-169.

BRUBAKER, C.E., & James, S. (1974). Injuries to runners. *Journal of Sports Medicine*, **2**, 189-199.

BUTLER, D.L., Grood, E.S., Noyes, F.R., & Zernicke, R.F. (1978). Biomechanics of ligaments and tendons. *Exercise and Sports Medicine Review*, **6**, 125-182.

CAPPOZZO, A. (1984). Gait analysis methodology. *Human Movement Science*, **3**, 27-50.

CATLIN, M.E., & Dressenhofer, R.F. (1979). Effects of shoe weight on the energy cost of running. *Medicine and Science in Sports and Exercise*, **11**, 80.

CAVAGNA, G.A. (1970). Elastic bounce of the body. *Journal of Applied Physiology*, **29**, 279-282.

CAVAGNA, G.A., & Margaria, R. (1964). Mechanical work in running. *Journal of Applied Physiology*, **39**, 174-179.

CAVANAGH, P.R. (1978a). A technique for averaging center of pressure paths from a force platform. *Journal of Biomechanics, Technical Note*, **11**, 487-491.

CAVANAGH, P.R. (1978b). Testing procedure. *Runner's World*, **10**, 70-80.

CAVANAGH, P.R. (1980). *The running shoe book*. Mountain View, CA: Anderson World, Inc.

CAVANAGH, P.R., Hennig, E.M., Bunch, R.P., & Macmillan, N.H. (1983). A new device for the measurement of pressure distribution inside the shoe. In H. Matsui & K. Kobayashi (Eds.), *Biomechanics VIII-B* (pp. 1089-1096). Champaign, IL: Human Kinetics Publishers.

CAVANAGH, P.R., Hinrichs, R.W., & Williams, K.R. (1980). Testing procedure for the 1981 *Runner's World* shoe survey. *Runner's World*, **15**, 33-49.

CAVANAGH, P.R., & Lafortune, M.A. (1980). Ground reaction forces in distance running. *Journal of Biomechanics*, **13**, 397-406.

CAVANAGH, P.R., & Michiyoshi, A.E. (1980). A technique for the display of pressure distribution beneath the foot. *Journal of Biomechanics*, **13**, 69-75.

CAVANAGH, P.R., Valiant, G.A., & Misevich, K.W. (1984). Biological aspects of modeling shoe/foot interaction during running. In E.C. Frederick (Ed.), *Sport shoes and playing surfaces* (pp. 24-46). Champaign, IL: Human Kinetics Publishers.

CAVANAGH, P.R., Williams, K.R., & Clarke, T.E. (1981). A comparison of ground reaction forces during walking barefoot and in shoes. In A. Morecki, K. Fidelus, K. Kedzior, & A. Wit (Eds.), *Biomechanics VII-B* (pp. 151-156). Baltimore: University Park Press.

CLANCY, W.G. (1982). Tendonitis and plantar fasciitis in runners. In R. D'Ambrosia and D. Drez (Eds). *Prevention and treatment of running injuries* (pp. 77-87). New Jersey: Slack.

CLARKE, T.E. (1980). *The pressure distribution under the foot during barefoot walking*. Unpublished doctoral dissertation. The Pennsylvania State University, University Park.

CLARKE, T.E., Frederick, E.C., & Cooper, L.B. (1982). The effects of shoe cushioning upon selected force and temporal parameters in running. *Medicine and Science in Sports and Exercise*, **14**, 144.

CLARKE, T.E., Frederick, E.C., & Cooper, L.B. (1983). Biomechanical measurement of running shoe cushioning properties. In B.M. Nigg & B.A. Kerr (Eds.), *Biomechanical aspects of sport shoes and playing surfaces* (pp. 25-33). Calgary: University Printing.

CLARKE, T.E., Frederick, E.C., & Hamill, C.L. (1983). The effects of shoe design parameters on rearfoot control in running. *Medicine and Science in Sports and Exercise*, **15**, 376-381.

CLARKE, T.E., Frederick, E.C., & Hamill, C.L. (1984). The study of rear foot movement in running. In E.C. Frederick (Ed.), *Sport shoes and playing surfaces* (pp. 166-189). Champaign, IL: Human Kinetics Publishers.

CLEMENT, D.B. (1982). Biomechanical analyses of overuse injuries in sports with experience of various foot corrections. *Proceedings of the National Seminar for Sport Injuries*, Turku, Finland.

CLEMENT, D.B., Taunton, J.E., Smart, G.W., & McNicol, K.L. (1981). A survey of overuse running injuries. *Physician Sports Medicine*, **9**, 47-58.

CLEMENT, D.B., Taunton, J.E., & Smart, G.W. (1984). Achilles tendinitis and peritendinitis: Etiology and treatment. *American Journal of Sports Medicine*, **12**, 179-184.

CLEMENT, D.B., Taunton, J.E., Wiley, J.P., Smart, G.W., & McNicol, K.L. (1982). Investigation of metabolic efficiency in runners with and without corrective orthotic devices. *International Journal of Sport Medicine*, **2**, 14-15.

CROWNINSHIELD, R.D., & Brand, R.A. (1981). A physiologically based criterion of muscle force prediction in locomotion. *Journal of Biomechanics*, **14**, 793-801.

D'AMBROSIA, R., & Douglas, R. (1982). Orthotics. In R. D'Ambrosia & D. Drez (Eds.), *Prevention and treatment of running injuries*. New Jersey: Slade.

DEBRUNNER, H.U. (1982). *Orthopaedic Diagnosis* (2nd ed.). New York: George Thieme.

DENOTH, J. (1977). Der einfluss des sportplatzbelages auf den menschlichen bewegungsapparat [The influence of playing surfaces on the locomotor system]. *Medita*, **9**, 164-167.

DENOTH, J. (1982). Biomechanische probleme der muskulaeren leistung [Biomechanical aspects of muscular performance]. In W. Groher & W. Noack (Eds.), *Sportliche Belastungsfaehigkeit des Haltungs—und Bewegungsapparates* (pp. 36-41). Stuttgart: Thieme.

DENOTH, J. (1983). A method to measure mechanical properties of soles and playing surfaces. In B.M. Nigg & B.A. Kerr (Eds.), *Biomechanical aspects of sport shoes and playing surfaces* (pp. 43-50). Calgary: University Printing.

DENOTH, J. (1985). The dynamic behavior of a three link model of the human body during impact with the ground. In D. Winter (Ed.), *Biomechanics IX-A* (pp. 102-106). Champaign, IL: Human Kinetics Publishers.

DENOTH, J., Gruber, K., Keepler, M., & Ruder, H. (in press). A model of the human body for a complete kinematic and dynamic description of a touch-down with high acceleration. In S. Perren (Ed.), *Biomechanics: Principles and Applications, Vol. 2*. Martinus Nijhoff Publishers.

DENOTH, J., Gruber, K., Keepler, M., & Ruder, H. (in press). Forces and torques during sport activities with high accelerations. In S. Perren (Ed.), *Biomechanics: Principles and Applications, Vol. 2*. Martinus Nijhoff Publishers.

DENOTH, J., Kaelin, X., & Stacoff, A. (in press). Schockabsorption beim jogging—materialtest contra versuchspersonentests [Cushioning during running—material tests contra subject tests]. *Sportmedizin.*

DENOTH, J., & Nigg, B.M. (1981). The influence of various sport floors on the load on the lower extremities. In A. Morecki, K. Fidelus, K. Kedizor, & A. Wit (Eds.), *Biomechanics VII-B* (pp. 100-105). Baltimore: University Park Press.

ELFTMAN, H. (1934). A cinematographic study of the distribution of pressure in the human foot. *Anatomical Record, 59*, 481-492.

FALSETTI, H.L., Burke, E.R., Feld, R., Frederick, E.C., & Ratering, C. (1983). Hematological variations after endurance running with hard and soft soled running shoes. *Physician & Sports Medicine, 11:8*, 118-127.

FREDERICK, E.C. (1983). Extrinsic biomechanical aids. In M.E. Williams (Ed.), *Ergogenic aids in sport* (pp. 323-339). Champaign, IL: Human Kinetics Publishers.

FREDERICK, E.C. (1983). Measuring the effects of shoes and surfaces on the economy of locomotion. In B.M. Nigg & B.A. Kerr (Eds.), *Biomechanical aspects of sport shoes and playing surfaces* (pp. 93-106). Calgary: University Printing.

FREDERICK, E.C., Clarke, T.E., & Hamill, C.L. (1984). The effect of running shoe design on shock attenuation. In E.C. Frederick (Ed.), *Sport shoes and playing surfaces* (pp. 190-198). Champaign, IL: Human Kinetics Publishers.

FREDERICK, E.C., Clarke, T.E., Larsen, J.L., & Cooper, L.B. (1983). The effects of shoe cushioning on the oxygen demands of running. In B.M. Nigg & B.A. Kerr (Eds.), *Biomechanical aspects of sport shoes and playing surfaces* (pp. 107-114). Calgary: University Printing.

FREDERICK, E.C., Hagy, J.L., & Mann, R.A. (1981). Prediction of vertical impact force during running. (abstract) *Journal of Biomechanics, 14*, 498.

FREDERICK, E.C., Howley, E.T., & Powers, S.K. (1980). Lower O_2 cost while running on air cushion type shoe. *Medicine and Science in Sports and Exercise, 12*, 81-82.

GERBER, H. (1982). A system for measuring dynamic pressure distribution under the human foot. *Journal of Biomechanics, Technical Note, 15:3*, 225-227.

GREENE, P.R., & McMahon, T.A. (1979). Reflex stiffness of man's anti-gravity muscles during knee bends while carrying extra weight. *Journal of Biomechanics, 12*, 881-891.

HATZE, H. (1981). *Myocybernetic control models of skeletal muscle.* Pretoria: University of South Africa.

HAY, J.G. (1981). *A bibliography of biomechanics literature (4th edition).* The University of Iowa.

HAYES, J., Smith, L., & Sanpietro, F. (1983). The effect of orthotics on the aerobic demands of running. *Medicine and Science in Sports and Exercise, 15*, 169.

HAYWARD, G.J. (1975). *Orthopaedic canvas shoe.* Utah, United States patent.

HENNING, E.M., Cavanagh, P.R., & Macmillan, N.H. (1983). Pressure distribution measurements by high precision piezoelectric ceramic force transducers. In H. Matsui & K. Kobayashi (Eds.), *Biomechanics VII-B* (pp. 1081-1088). Champaign, IL: Human Kinetics Publishers.

HESS, H., & Hort, W. (1973). Erhoehte verletzungsgefahr beim leichtathletiktraining auf kunststoffboeden [Increased danger of injuries on artificial surfaces during training in track and field]. *Sportarzt und Sportmedizin, 12*, 282-285.

HLAVAC, H.F. (1977). *The foot book*. Mountain View, CA: Anderson World Inc.

HILL, A.V. (1970). *First and last experiments in muscle mechanics*. Cambridge University Press.

HORT, W. (1976). Ursachen, klinik, therapie und prophylaxe der schaeden auf leichtathletik-kunststoffbahnen [Origin, clinical treatment, therapy and prevention of injuries on artificial track and field surfaces]. *Leistungssport*, **1**, 48052.

HORT, W. (1979). Der sportschuh auf modernen kunststoffbelaegen und seine bedeutung fuer die aufrechterhaltung der leistungsfaehigkeit [The sportshoe on modern artificial surfaces and its significance for the maintenance of the capacity of performance]. *Leistungssport*, **9**, 206-209.

HUBBARD, R.P., & Soutas-Little, R.W. (1984). Mechanical properties of human tendon and their age dependence. *Journal of Biomechanical Engineering*, **106**, 144-150.

INMAN, V.T. (1976). *The joints of the ankle*. Baltimore: Williams & Wilkins Co.

JACKSON, D.W. (1978). Shinsplints: an update. *Physician Sports Medicine*, **6**, 49-68.

JAMES, S., Bates, B., & Osternig, L. (1978). Injuries in runners. *American Journal of Sports Medicine*, **6**, 40-50.

KAELIN, X., Denoth, J., Stacoff, A., & Stuessi, E. (in press). Cushioning during running—material tests contra subject tests. In S. Perren (Ed.), *Biomechanics: Principles and Applications, Vol. 2*. Martinus Nijhoff Publishers.

KAELIN, X., Unold, E., Stuessi, E., & Stacoff, A. (1985). Interindividual and intraindividual variabilities in running. In D. Winter (Ed.), *Biomechanics IX-B* (pp. 356-360). Champaign, IL: Human Kinetics Publishers.

KOLITZUS, H.J. (1984). Functional standards for playing surfaces. In E.C. Frederick (Ed.), *Sport shoes and playing surfaces* (pp. 98-118). Champaign, IL: Human Kinetics Publishers.

KOMI, P.V. (1983). Biomechanical features of running with special emphasis on load characteristics and mechanical efficiency. In B.M. Nigg & B.A. Kerr (Eds.), *Biomechanical aspects of sport shoes and playing surfaces* (pp. 123-134). Calgary: University Printing.

KRISSOFF, W.B., & Ferris, W.D. (1979). Runner's injuries. *The Physician and Sports Medicine*, **7**:12, 55-64.

KUNZ, H. (1978). Das sprungkrafttraining [The training of take-off forces]. *Schweizer Turnen und Leichtathletik*, **15**, 12-14.

LANGE, F. (1914). *Orthopaedisches lehrbuch*. Jena: Fischer.

LANYON, L.E., Hampson, W.G.J., Goodship, A.E., & Shah, J.S. (1975). Bone deformation recorded in vivo from strain gauges attached to the human tibial shaft. *Acta Orthopaedical Scandinavica*, **46**, 256-268.

LANZ, T., & Wachsmuth, W. (1972). *Praktische anatomy* [Practical anatomy]. Berlin: Springer Verlag.

LEACH, R. (1982). Running injuries of the knee. In R. D'Ambrosia & D. Drez (Eds.), *Prevention and treatment of running injuries* (pp. 55-75). New Jersey: Slade.

LIGHT, L.H., McLellan, G.E., & Klenerman, L. (1980). Skeletal transients on heel strike in normal walking with different footwear. *Journal of Biomechanics*, **13**, 477-480.

LORD, M. (1981). Foot pressure measurement: A review of methodology. *Journal of Biomedical Engineering*, **3**, 91-99.

LUETHI, S.M. (1983). *Biomechanical analysis of short term pain and injuries in tennis.* Unpublished doctoral dissertation. University of Calgary.

LUETHI, S.M., Nigg, B.M., & Bahlsen, H.A. (1984). The influence of varying shoe sole stiffnesses on impact forces in running. *Proceedings of the Annual Conference of the Canadian Society of Biomechanics,* Human Locomotion III.

McMAHON, T.A., & Green, P.R. (1979). The influence of trade compliance on running. *Journal of Biomechanics,* **12**, 893-904.

MANN, R.A. (1982). Biomechanics of running. In R. D'Ambrosia & D. Drez (Eds.), *Prevention and treatment of running injuries.* New Jersey: Slade.

MARCUS, B. (1983). *The influence of footwear and surfaces on performance and injury potential in running.* Unpublished doctoral dissertation. Imperial College, University of London.

MASSART, R. (1938). *Pratique orthopedic* [Practical orthopaedics]. Paris: Amadee Legrand.

MISEVICH, K.W., & Cavanagh, P.R. (1984). Material aspects of modelling shoe/foot interaction. In E.C. Frederick (Ed.), *Sport shoes and playing surfaces* (pp. 47-75). Champaign, IL: Human Kinetics Publishers.

MIURA, M., Miyashita, M., Matsui, H., & Sodeyama, H. (1974). Photographic method of analysing the pressure distribution of the foot against the ground. In R.C. Nelson & C.A. Morehouse (Eds.), *Biomechanics IV* (pp. 482-487). Baltimore: University Park Press.

MORRISON, J.B. (1969). Bioengineering analysis of force actions transmitted by the knee joint. *Biomedical Engineering,* **4**, 164-170.

MORRISON, J.B. (1970). The mechanics of the knee joint in relation to normal walking. *Journal of Biomechanics,* **3**, 51-61.

NICOL, K., & Hennig, E.M. (1976). Time dependent method for measuring force distribution using a flexible mat as a capacitor. In P.V. Komi (Ed.), *Biomechanics V-B* (pp. 433-440). Baltimore: University Park Press.

NIGG, B.M. (1980). Biomechanische ueberlegungen zur belastung des bewegungs-apparates [Biomechanical considerations on the loading of the musculo-skeletal system]. In H. Cotta, H. Krahl, & K. Steinbrueck (Eds.), *Die Belastungstoleranz des Bewegungsapparates* (pp. 44-54). Stuttgart: Thieme Verlag.

NIGG, B.M. (1983). External force measurements with sport shoes and playing surfaces. In B.M. Nigg & B.A. Kerr (Eds.), *Biomechanical aspects of sport shoes and playing surfaces* (pp. 11-23). Calgary: University Printing.

NIGG, B.M., & Denoth, J. (1980). *Sportplatzbelaege* [Playing surfaces]. Juris Verlag, Zurich.

NIGG, B.M., Denoth, J., Kerr, B.A., Luethi, S.M., Smith, D., & Stacoff, A. (1984). Load, sport shoes and playing surfaces. In E.C. Frederick (Ed.), *Sport shoes and playing surfaces* (pp. 1-23). Champaign, IL: Human Kinetics Publishers.

NIGG, B.J., Denoth, J., & Neukomm, P.A. (1981). Quantifying the load on the human body: Problems and some possible solutions. In A. Morecki, K. Fidelus, K. Kedzior, & A. Wit (Eds.), *Biomechanics VII* (pp. 88-99). Baltimore: University Park Press.

NIGG, B.M., Denoth, J., Neukomm, P.A., & Segesser, B. (1978). *Biomechanische aspekte zu sportplatzbelaegen* [Biomechanical aspects on playing surfaces]. Juris Verlag, Zurich.

NIGG, B.M., Eberle, G., Frey, D., Luethi, S.M., Segesser, B., & Weber, B. (1978). Gait analysis and sport shoe construction. In E. Asmussen & K. Joergensen (Eds.), *Biomechanics VI-A* (pp. 303-309). Baltimore: University Park Press.

NIGG, B.M., Eberle, G., Frey, D., & Segesser, B. (1977). Biomechanische analyse von fussinsuffizienzen [Biomechanical analysis of foot insufficiencies]. *Medizinisch-Orthopaedische Technik,* **97,** 178-180.

NIGG, B.M., Eberle, G., Frey, D., Segesser, B., & Weber, B. (1977). Bewegungs-analyse fuer schuhkorrekturen [Movement analysis for shoe corrections]. *Medita,* **9a,** 160-163.

NIGG, B.M., & Luethi, S.M. (1980). Bewegungsanalysen beim laufschuh [Movement analysis for running shoes]. *Sportwissenschaft,* **3,** 309-320.

NIGG, B.M., Luethi, S.M., Segesser, B., Stacoff, A., Guidon, H.W., & Schneider, A. (1982). *Sportschuhkorrekturen: Ein biomechanischer vergleich von drei verschiedenen sportschuhkorrekturen* [Sport shoe support inlays: A biomechanical comparison of three different types of arch support]. *Z. Orthop.,* **120,** 34-39.

NIGG, B.M., Luethi, S.M., Stacoff, A., & Segesser, B. (1984). Biomechanical effects of pain and sport shoe corrections. *The Australian Journal of Science and Medicine,* **16,** 10-16.

NIGG, B.M., Neukomm, P.A., Spirig, J., & Unold, E. (1974). Die belastung des menschlichen bewegungsapparates bei sportlicher betaetigung [Load on the musculo-skeletal system in various sport activities]. *NZZ: Forschung und Technik,* **466,** 79-82.

NIGG, B.M., Neukomm, P.A., & Unold, E. (1974). Biomechanik und sport [Biomechanics and sport]. *Orthopaede,* **3,** 140-147.

PAGLIANO, J., & Jackson, D. (1980). The ultimate study of running injuries. *Runner's World,* **11,** 42-50.

PAUL, J.P. (1965). Bioengineering studies of the forces transmitted by joints. In R.M. Kennedy (Ed.), *Engineering analysis, biomechanics and related bioengineering topics* (pp. 369-380). Oxford: Pergamon Press.

PAUL, J.P. (1967). Forces transmitted by joints in the human body. *Proceedings of the Institute of Mechanical Engineering,* **181**(3J), 8. Paper presented at the Institute of Mechanical Engineering Symposium in Lubrication and Wear and Artificial Human Joints, London.

PAUWELS, F. (1973). *Atlas zur biomechanik der gesunden und kranken huefte* [Atlas on the biomechanics of the healthy and ill hip]. Berlin: Springer Verlag.

PEDOTTI, A., Krishnan, V.V., & Starke, L. (1978). Optimization of muscle-force sequencing in human locomotion. *Mathematics and Biosciences,* **38,** 57-76.

PERKINS, P.J., & Wilson, M.P. (1983). Slip resistance testing of shoes—new developments. *Ergonomics,* **26,** 73-82.

PIERRYNOWSKI, M.R. (1982). *A physiological model for the solution of individual muscle force during normal human walking.* Unpublished doctoral dissertation. Simon Fraser University.

PROCTER, P. (1980). *Ankle joint biomechanics.* Unpublished doctoral dissertation. University of Strathclyde.

PROCTER, P., Berme, N., & Paul, J.P. (1981). Ankle joint biomechanics. In A. Morecki, K. Fidelus, K. Kedizor, & A. Wit (Eds.), *Biomechanics VII-A* (pp. 52-56). Baltimore: University Park Press.

PROKOP, L., & Haberl, R. (1972, 1973). Die auswirkungen von kunststoffbahnen auf den bewegungsapparat [The effect of artificial tracks on the human body]. *Oesterreichisches Journal fuer Sportmedizin,* **2** (1972), **3** (1972), **4** (1972), **1** (1973).

PROKOP, L. (1976). Sportmedizinische probleme der kunststoffbelaege [Sports medical problems of artificial surfaces]. *Sportstaettenbau und Baederanlagen,* **4**, 1175-1181.

RABL, C.R.H. (1975). *Orthopaedie des fusses* [Orthopedics of the foot]. Enke Verlag, Stuttgart: 5. Auflage.

RADIN, E.L., Orr, R.B., Kelman, J.L., Paul, I.L., & Rose, R.M. (1982). Effect of prolonged walking on concrete on the knees of sheep. *Journal of Biomechanics,* **15**, 487-492.

RADIN, E.L., Parker, H.G., Pugh, G.V., Steinberg, R.S., Paul, I.L., & Rose, R.M. (1973). Response of joints to impact loading. *Journal of Biomechanics,* **6**, 51-57.

RHEINSTEIN, D.J., Morehouse, C.A., & Niebel, B.W. (1978). Effects of traction of outsole composition and hardnesses of basketball shoes and three types of playing surfaces. *Medicine and Science in Sports,* **10**, 282-288.

ROMANES, A.J. (1976). *Cunningham's manual of practical anatomy,* 14th Edition. London: Oxford University Press.

ROSSI, W.A. (1980). The last, heart of the shoe. *Journal of American Podiatry Association,* **70**, 533-534.

SCHLAEPFER, F., Unold, E., & Nigg, B.M. (1983). The frictional characteristics of tennis shoes. In B.M. Nigg & B.A. Kerr (Eds.), *Biomechanical aspects of sport shoes and playing surfaces* (pp. 153-160). Calgary: University Printing.

SCHMIDTBLEICHER, D. (1980). *Innervationsverhalten bei landungen auf unterschiedlich harten matten* [Muscle inervation during landing on mats with different hardness]. Paper presented at the Symposium of the ITB in Heidelberg.

SEGESSER, B. (1970). *Sportschaeden durch ungeeignete boeden in sportanlagen* [Sport injuries as a consequence of unsuitable surfaces]. Arztdienst, ETS Magglingen.

SEGESSER, B. (1976). Die belastung des bewegungsappartes auf kunststoffboeden [Loading of the musculo-skeletal system on artificial surfaces]. *Sportstaettenbau und Baederanlagen,* **4**, 1183-1194.

SEGESSER, B., & Nigg, B.M. (1980). Insertionstendinosen am schienbein, achillodynie und ueberlastungsfolgen am fuss—aetiologie, biomechanik, therapeutische moeglichkeiten [Tibial insertion tendinoses, achillodynia and damage to overuse of the foot—etiology, biomechanics, therapy]. *Orthopaede,* **9**, 207-214.

SEGESSER, B., Nigg, B.M., & Morell, F. (1980). Achillodynie und tibiale insertionstendinosen [Achillodynia and tibial insertion tendinoses]. *Med. u. Sport,* **29**, 79-83.

SEGESSER, B., Ruepp, R., & Nigg, B.M. (1978). Indikation, technik und fehlermoeglichkeit einer sportschuhkorrektur [Indication, error possibilities and techniques of a sport shoe correction]. *Orthopaedische Praxis,* **11**, 834-837.

SEGESSER, B., & Stacoff, A. (1981). Verletzungsprophylaxe durch geeignetes sportschuhwerk [Injury prophylaxes through suited sportshoes]. *Orthopaedie Schuhtechnik,* **7**, 308-315.

SEGESSER, B., & Stacoff, A. (1982a). Jeder laufschuh ist ein kompromiss [Each running shoe is a compromise]. *Sporterziehung in der Schule,* **5,6**, 25-27.

SEGESSER, B., & Stacoff, A. (1982b). Tibial insertion tendinoses, achillodynia and damage due to overuse of the foot—etiology, biomechanics and therapy. *Proceedings of the National Seminar for Sport Injuries*. Turku, Finland.

SEGESSER, B., Stacoff, A., & Nigg, B.M. (1983). Die belastbarkeit der sprunggelenke aus biomechanisch-klinischer sicht. *Medizin und Sport 23*, **H1-3**, 9-13.

SEIREG, A., & Arvikar, R.J. (1973). A mathematical model for evaluation of forces in lower extremities of the musculo-skeletal system. *Journal of Biomechanics*, **6**, 313-326.

SEIREG, A., & Arvikar, R.J. (1975). The prediction of muscular load sharing and joint forces in the lower extremities during walking. *Journal of Biomechanics*, **8**, 89-102.

SMART, G.W., Taunton, J.E., & Clement, D.B. (1980). Achilles tendon disorders in runners—a review. *Medicine and Science in Sports and Exercise*, **4**, 231-243.

STACOFF, A. (1984). Schuhtests. In: *Biomechanische aspekte zu sportschuhen und tennisschleaegern* [Biomechanical aspects of sportshoes and tennis rackets]. Zurich: Labor fuer Biomechanik.

STACOFF, A., & Kaelin, X. (1983). Pronation and sportshoe design. In B.M. Nigg & B.A. Kerr (Eds.), *Biomechanical aspects of sport shoes and playing surfaces* (pp. 143-151). Calgary: University Printing.

STACOFF, A., & Stuessi, E. (in press). Biomechanische aspekte zur belastung der sprunggelenke [Biomechanical aspects of load at the ankle joints]. *Vortrag am 1. Basler Symposium fuer Sportmedizin.*

STACOFF, A., Stuessi, E., & Sonderegger, D. (1985). Lateral stability of sportshoes. In D. Winter (Ed.), *Biomechanics IX-B* (pp. 139-143). Champaign, IL: Human Kinetics Publishers.

STUESSI, E., Aebersold, P., & Debrunner, H.U. (1978). Darstellung des ganges durch vierdmensionale vektoren [Illustration of gait by 4-D vectors]. *Biomedizinische Technik*, **23**, 25.

SUBOTNICK, S.I. (1979). *Cures for common running injuries*. Mountain View, CA: Anderson World, Inc.

SUBOTNICK, S.I. (1981). The flat foot. *Physician and Sports Medicine*, **9**, 85-91.

TANNER, J.M. (1964). *The physique of the Olympic athlete*. London: Allen and Unwin Ltd.

TIEGERMANN, V. (1983). Reaction forces and EMG activity in fast sideward movements. In B.M. Nigg & B.A. Kerr (Eds.), *Biomechanical aspects of sport shoes and playing surfaces* (pp. 83-90). Calgary: University Printing.

UNOLD, E. (1974). Erschuetterungsmessungen beim gehen und laufen auf verschiedenen unterlagen mit verschiedenem schuhwerk [Acceleration measurements during walking and running on various surfaces with different shoes]. *Jugend und Sport*, **8**, 289-292.

VAN GHELUWE, B., Deporte, E., & Hebbelinck, M. (1983). Frictional forces and torques of soccer shoes on artifical turf. In B.M. Nigg & B.A. Kerr (Eds.), *Biomechanical aspects of sport shoes and playing surfaces* (pp. 161-168). Calgary: University Printing.

VOLOSHIN, A., & Wosk, J. (1982). An in vivo study of low back pain and shock absorption in the human locomotor system. *Journal of Biomechanics*, **15**, 21-27.

VON MEYER, H. (1858). *Die richtige gestalt der schuhe* [The correct form of shoes]. Zurich: Meyer and Zoeller.

WILLIAMS, K.R. (1982). Non-saggital plane movements and forces during distance running. *Proceedings of the Sixth Annual Conference of the ASB.*

WINTER, D.A. (1983). Moments of force and mechanical power in jogging. *Journal of Biomechanics, 16,* 91-97.

WINTER, D.A. (1984). Kinematic and kinetic patterns in human gait: Variability and compensating effects. *Human Movement Science, 3,* 51-76.

YAMADA, H. (1970). *Strength of biological materials.* Baltimore: F. Gaynor Evans, Williams, & Wilkins.

ZAMOSKY, I. (1964, Fall). Shoe modifications in lower extremity orthotics. *Bulletin of Prosthetics Research.*

Index